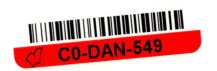

Searching *for* Health

A JOHNS HOPKINS PRESS HEALTH BOOK

Searching *for* Health

The Smart Way to Find Information
Online and Put It to Use

KAPIL PARAKH, MD, PhD

with **ANNA DIRKSEN**

Johns Hopkins University Press | *Baltimore*

Note to the Reader: This book is not meant to substitute for medical care, and treatment should not be based solely on its contents. Instead, treatment must be developed in a dialogue between the individual and his or her physician. The book has been written to help with that dialogue.

While this is a book about health, it does not provide medical advice, nor does it substitute for medical advice or services provided by a trained medical professional. The views expressed by the authors and publishers do not represent those of Google, Alphabet, its subsidiaries, or any other entity with which the authors may be affiliated. The information within this book is provided for educational purposes without any representations or warranties, express or implied. The authors and publishers specifically disclaim any responsibility for any liability, loss, or risk incurred as a consequence (directly or indirectly) of the use of this book.

© 2021 Johns Hopkins University Press
All rights reserved. Published 2021
Printed in the United States of America on acid-free paper
9 8 7 6 5 4 3 2 1

Reproduction in whole or in part without written permission from
Johns Hopkins University Press is strictly prohibited.

Johns Hopkins University Press
2715 North Charles Street
Baltimore, Maryland 21218-4363
www.press.jhu.edu

Library of Congress Cataloging-in-Publication Data

Names: Parakh, Kapil, 1978– author. | Dirksen, Anna, 1976– contributor.
Title: Searching for health : the smart way to find information online and put it to use /
    Kapil Parakh, MD, PhD ; with Anna Dirksen.
Description: Baltimore : Johns Hopkins University Press, [2021] | Series: A Johns
    Hopkins press health book | Includes bibliographical references and index.
Identifiers: LCCN 2020020191 | ISBN 9781421440279 (hardcover) | ISBN 9781421440286
    (paperback) | ISBN 9781421440293 (ebook)
Subjects: LCSH: Medicine, Popular—Computer network resources. | Medicine—
    Computer network resources. | Medical care—Computer network resources. |
    Consumer education.
Classification: LCC RC82 .P377 2021 | DDC 610.285—dc23
LC record available at https://lccn.loc.gov/2020020191

A catalog record for this book is available from the British Library.

*Special discounts are available for bulk purchases of this book. For more information, please
contact Special Sales at specialsales@jh.edu.*

Johns Hopkins University Press uses environmentally friendly book materials, including
recycled text paper that is composed of at least 30 percent post-consumer waste, whenever
possible.

To my dad, who will never know how much he inspired me, and to my family, friends, and mentors, who have tirelessly supported and encouraged me.
Thank you.
Kapil Parakh

For Matthew and our girls, Neala and Willa
Anna Dirksen

Contents

List of Worksheets

How to Use This Book

When we started writing this book, our goal was to give readers a set of tips to search for health information online: how to craft a powerful search string, how to accurately read search results, and how to find detailed medical information. But as our writing unfolded, so did the scope of the book itself.

Every health journey is unique, which means that most of us travel down many paths in order to find the health information we need. In some cases, our best sources of information are online. In other cases, we may need to turn to pharmacists, patient advocates, or integrative medicine providers to find the answers we need. And through it all, we need to keep communicating what we learn with the doctors and nurses who traditionally manage our care so that everyone is working together toward improving our health.

To address these needs most effectively, we chose to organize the book around each component of a person's health journey. The book starts with the first signs of illness and then goes through the process of getting a diagnosis and deciding on treatment options, including surgery, medications, and lifestyle changes. We also talk about the tough decisions people often have to make when their health challenges become critical, including choices around end-of-life care.

Some readers may prefer to read this book cover to cover. Those wrestling with a specific phase of the journey may want to dive directly into the chapter most relevant to them. To help those going straight to a specific chapter, we have cross-referenced related materials in other parts of the book to make it easier to find all the relevant content.

In some chapters, we include a section called "Think Like Your Doctor" that provides a glimpse into clinical reasoning and offers practical tips based on a health care provider's approach to help you take better control of your health.* Appearing at the end of most chapters are checklists, forms, or resources that expand on these tips and can be used separately from the chapters to help you record important medical information and think through decisions.

The personal stories we feature in the book are from people we met through our research and from Dr. Parakh's clinical experience. In some cases, we feature people who shared their story with the public prior to us writing the book. Each story illustrates how challenging it is to make important decisions about your health or the health of those you love. Each one also demonstrates how it can be done successfully.

As we wrapped up the writing of our book, news of a novel coronavirus pandemic was just beginning to break. Health care systems across the world were struggling to cope with a surge in demand. In places like Spain, Italy, and here in the United States, people were being asked to stay home for the safety of all. In such trying times, with the fragility of our health care systems exposed, it is more important than ever to feel empowered to find the health information you need and to advocate for yourself with your health care providers. We hope that this book becomes a well-thumbed resource on your path to better health in both the best and worst of times.

---

* We recognize that there are many providers that deliver health care. At times we use the word *doctor* as a catchall term for the wider group of providers and specialists.

Searching *for* Health

Prologue

I have long believed in the power of knowledge to improve health. From managing chronic disease to combating epidemics, patient education and empowerment can have a tremendous impact on reducing suffering and saving lives. But, as a practicing cardiologist, I often see patients who are overwhelmed by their diagnosis and unable to process all the information we discuss during our short office visits.

Like most doctors, my biggest challenge is lack of time. Clinic visits have become ever shorter because of documentation requirements, clunky electronic medical records, red tape, and shrinking reimbursements from insurance companies. Other challenges abound. Sometimes patients come with misperceptions that need to be addressed. Other times there are health literacy and numeracy barriers. Sometimes there are cultural beliefs that have to be placed into context. The list goes on.

Over the course of my career, I have tried different approaches to overcome these challenges and help patients process the vast amount of information that they have to navigate. As a resident, I would print out detailed education material for patients and their families. As a fellow, I would schedule patients more frequently and give out information in smaller, more digestible chunks. As a cardiologist at Johns Hopkins Bayview Medical

Center, I created a comprehensive patient education program. At Google, I helped build products that made health information more accessible for over a billion users.

Along the way, I have become absolutely convinced of the tremendous potential of the internet. It has become a valuable source of useful information for me both professionally and personally. My father suffered from dementia since he was just fifty-seven years old. In the early years, he had subtle signs of the disease. Over time, his condition relentlessly worsened until he could no longer recognize me or my brother, and it became near impossible for my mother to continue caring for him at home. Ultimately, we were faced with the decision of whether he should be moved to a long-term care facility. Initially, my mother and our extended family resisted the idea. I struggled with the choice as well. But after looking online and speaking to experts, the health information in his case was clear — my father would soon need very specialized care that could not be made available at home. So, we chose the path that was the best for my father's health, without feeling guilty about our decision despite how hard it stung. In the ensuing eighteen months, the facility took wonderful care of him until his passing. I will forever be grateful that he had the support he needed in his final months.

Even with my expertise, it was incredibly difficult for me to navigate that experience. I realized that there could be real value in a book that could help people make more informed health decisions. As I was thinking through the idea, my wife suggested that I reach out to our friend, and now my coauthor, Anna. In speaking with her, it became clear that Anna's perspective and practical approach were the ideal counterbalance to the technical constructs I was exploring. Together, we could craft a narrative that was practical, grounded in science, and yet accessible to a wide audience.

This book is the result of our collaboration. It seeks to bridge the chasm between the valuable health information that exists online and the person on the other end of the search box, struggling to find the right information for them. We believe the tools provided in this book will empower people to collaborate more effectively with their health care providers and make better decisions about their health. Ultimately, we hope the result is that more people live a healthier and happier life.

Kapil Parakh, MD, PhD

I was five months pregnant when my husband and I moved to Tokyo in the fall of 2011. We had no family there, few friends, and little understanding of the nuances of the culture. We were fortunate to find a British clinic with doctors and nurses who worked in English during all our prenatal visits. Our daughter arrived a few months later.

My husband returned to the clinic just after our daughter's first birthday, for a hemorrhoid, he thought. His doctor removed it, took a biopsy, and then emailed a week later to say that the pathologist had found "significant abnormalities." I recall little from our next appointment. What sticks out was the doctor's use of the word *carcinoma*.

We spent the next six months shuttling to appointments, chemotherapy, and radiation. All the cancer specialists, nurses, and technicians we met during treatment were Japanese. Few of them spoke English. We asked ourselves over and over whether we understood what they were trying to explain to us, and we worried about where our decisions might take us.

So, like everyone else in this situation, we turned to the internet. We opened our laptops every day and searched. What are the side effects of this type of chemotherapy? Will we be able to have another child? How does radiation affect the skin?

We found a lot of information that reassured us. But every revelation prompted more questions. I joined a Facebook group that gave me more insight into what my husband was going through. I also found site after site that sent me into a panic. At the worst of times, what I read made me second-guess our choices and wonder whether the treatment was doing more harm than good.

You may have picked up this book because you've felt your own misgivings about a choice you were making about your health. The internet provides us with ever more opportunities to understand our health. We can find causes of our symptoms, methods to manage them and, in the best-case scenarios, treatments that we can try with the support of our doctors. We can also confuse ourselves, jump to conclusions, and misdiagnose the cause of our discomfort.

When Kapil approached me about this book, I wasn't convinced. I asked him who would read a book instead of just typing "strange rash on arm" into a search box. Kapil is a cardiologist who, through his work with Google, has made it easier for all of us to search for what might ail us. He helped me remember my own odyssey and the many times I felt lost.

My hope is that this book will provide you with the support I searched for myself when my husband and I were going through our most challenging moments. I hope it leaves you feeling confident and reassured about the decisions you make along your own journey to wellness.

Anna Dirksen, MSc

1 | The First Signs of Illness

The episode started with a fever, as many illnesses do. Xavier Downton was four years old and had just finished his first week of kindergarten. His mother, Rachelle, had taken him to the rink to watch his brother's hockey practice. She put her hand up to Xavier's face and noticed he felt hot.

Rachelle took her boys to their home near Ottawa, Ontario, Canada, after practice and checked Xavier's temperature. It was high, but not high enough to raise any alarms. She figured it was a cold he had picked up at school. So, she gave him some medicine and helped him to bed.

Xavier still had a fever the next day, but it hadn't gotten any worse. He complained about some aches. Still, he was in a good mood. And he had not lost his appetite. "We were asking ourselves, 'Should we go to the clinic, or not?'" Rachelle said. "But I was looking up the flu online and he had all the symptoms. It was Labor Day weekend, and I thought we'd spend hours waiting in the emergency room only to have them send us home. He was hydrated. He was eating. And he had no other signs like vomiting or diarrhea. So, we decided it was better to stay home."

By Monday evening, at the end of the long weekend, Rachelle and her husband were feeling good about their decision. Xavier's fever was gone, and it seemed as though the illness was running its course. Rachelle settled into bed beside Xavier, dozing off beside him as he slept. A little while later, he rolled over, waking her up. She checked him again and noticed something strange. His right arm was limp as he rolled onto his side. She wondered if she was imagining it, but there was clearly something wrong.

A similar story was unfolding more than a thousand miles away in Minnesota. Mehdi and Victoria Ayouche's five-year-old daughter, Sophia, had developed a fever and some aches. They assumed she had a cold. They, too, tried to ride it out. When Sophia didn't get better, they took her to a doctor. The doctor diagnosed her with strep throat and sent her home with a course of antibiotics. A few days later, her arm went limp. Now, Mehdi was hovering over her as doctors at a children's hospital in St. Paul examined her.

After a range of tests and numerous misdiagnoses, both Sophia and Xavier were diagnosed with acute flaccid myelitis (AFM), a polio-like disease that popped up in the autumn of 2018 in headline after headline. AFM is a rare but serious condition that affects the nervous system, specifically the gray matter of the spinal cord. The disease can cause muscles and reflexes to become weak.[1] More than 90 percent of those with AFM start out with a mild respiratory illness or fever. But the virus persists, the illness evolves, and the person's symptoms become progressively worse.

Researchers are striving to find out more about AFM, but they have limited data to work with. In 2018, there were fewer than two hundred confirmed cases of AFM across the United States. Yet, if you were to look online or watch the news at the time, you would have thought that the disease was the next global pandemic. "An echo of polio: AFM paralyzes children and terrifies parents," reported the *Chicago Tribune*[2] "Polio-like illness is on the rise," according to NBC News.[3]

Parents like Rachelle Downton and Mehdi Ayouche took to the media to share any information they could. "My goal was to calm parents but also to let them know what to look out for," Rachelle said. "I wanted them to know that this can happen to anybody but it's very,

very rare. I wanted them to be on the lookout for those signs, but I also didn't want them to panic for no reason."

Rachelle, Mehdi, and other parents who told their stories alerted people to the disease. But not everyone knew what to do with the information. Between September and October 2018, online searches for "polio-like virus" and "AFM" increased a hundred-fold. Worried parents and grandparents were posting messages on Facebook and elsewhere asking how long they should monitor a child who had the flu and when they should see a doctor. People were posting videos on YouTube claiming that routine childhood vaccinations caused the disease and hyping alternative treatments as cures. Many parents were understandably confused.

The Trouble with the Internet

Think of any illness—breast cancer, heart disease, diabetes—and the first thing many of us do when confronted with the potential of having such an illness is to go online. Recent studies suggest that when Americans have questions about their health, they turn first to the internet.[4] A study out of Australia found that more than one-third of ER patients searched their symptoms online before deciding whether to go to the hospital.[5] Other studies have confirmed the trend.[6,7,8]

Given the time and resources required to visit a doctor's office or urgent care clinic, it makes sense that more people are turning to the internet instead. But this approach carries a risk. A survey of two thousand Americans suggested that three-quarters of people whose first step was to search their symptoms online ended up worrying more because of what they found.[9] Forty-three percent of respondents said that, after their search, they were convinced that they had a serious disease, which, in fact, they did not end up having.

Many of us go online to look for answers to every question we might have, from how to register to vote to the best place to eat dinner on a Friday night. In doing that with our health, many of us end up misinformed. The problem may lie in our approach. Each of us has consciously or subconsciously developed a process for our searches, a routine those in the technology space call the *user journey*.

For most users, their journey starts with either a specific search such as "best Italian restaurant near me" or a broad one such as "best place to eat in Boston." We refine our queries using criteria that are important to us to get to the answers we're looking for. This user journey has become so commonplace that most people follow some variation of it without giving it any thought. But, when it comes to your health, this approach may be ineffective.

Research suggests that searches for health information are distinctive for a number of reasons. First, users are often unfamiliar with health care language and are likely to conduct an initial search without well-defined keywords.[10] As a result, their search is often exploratory rather than focused, with users learning more as they go and adapting their search terms as needed. Some of the information a person learns during a search can alarm them. A Microsoft study showed that people often start by searching for common, relatively innocuous symptoms, then end up reading content on rare and serious conditions.[11]

Doctors, nurses, and other health care providers undergo years of training. Most of them are able to quickly process the available information in relation to a patient's symptoms. However, the average person going online does not have that expertise. The majority of people surveyed in a study from Australia said that they wanted more guidance to help find the right health information on the internet.[12]

Our book gives you a framework that you can use whenever you go online to look for answers about your health. The approach is guided by research studies and publications from credible institutions such as the National Institutes of Health and the National Academy of Medicine. However, few studies have examined how to effectively navigate health information online.[13] We have gone beyond such research and have sought inspiration from the frameworks that doctors use in practice every day.

The goal is not to replace your doctor but to provide a set of tools that you can apply to your searches to improve your ability to find the right information to guide decisions about your health. Studies suggest that the internet can improve outcomes by enhancing our understanding of health issues, increasing our belief in ourselves and our ability to take control of our health, and refining our interactions with the health care system.[14] We include recommendations on how to communicate productively with your health care providers and become an active and engaged member of your health care team.

Where It All Begins

Many people start exploring questions related to their health when a symptom first occurs. You have a fever, a nagging headache, or a rash and try to figure out what's wrong. For the parents of the children affected by AFM, their journey started with what seemed like the first sign of the flu: a mild fever.

Many parents in that moment are tempted to go online. That response, however, comes with risk. The ready availability of a search box, which is supposed to improve access to information, is the very thing that could lead you astray. In the early 1900s, neurologist George Lincoln Walton noticed an odd behavior among medical students learning about a new disease: "The knowledge that pneumonia produces pain in a certain spot leads to a concentration of attention upon that region which causes any sensation there to give alarm. The mere knowledge of the location of the appendix transforms the most harmless sensations in that region into symptoms of serious menace."

This phenomenon is more commonly known as *medical students' disease* or *intern's syndrome*. Some students, as they learn about a new condition, begin to experience the symptoms of the disease because they pay more attention to that part of their body or those sensations. The average person searching for their symptoms online experiences this too.

Let's say you go online because you notice an ache in your stomach. The search results pop up. Is it a burning sensation? Does it often occur after you eat? You hadn't really thought about it before but now that you're reading these articles, you start to think that maybe your stomach does feel a bit like it's burning. At your next meal, you pay attention to the area, and it's true — it does hurt after you eat. Your understanding of your symptom has shifted without your pain actually changing. This happens to us all the time because symptoms are dynamic and dependent on circumstances. Feeling tired at 4 p.m. near the end of a workday is one thing. Feeling tired after eight hours of sleep on a relaxing weekend is something else.

Our memory of when symptoms occur, and their intensity, is usually foggy. Researchers in the United Kingdom asked more than one hundred people to keep health diaries for three months.[15] The respondents recorded the frequency, duration, and severity of health events, including symptoms. When the three months were up, they turned in their diaries. Then, the researchers asked each respondent to describe their health history over that period. On average, participants forgot more than half of the health events that they had experienced.

Think Like Your Doctor: Using a Symptom Tracker

The story above underscores the unreliability of memory. So, think like your doctor and write down your symptoms from the beginning. If your daughter complains of a stomachache, write down what she is feeling, what she was feeling or doing before the symptom started, and how those feelings change over time. We recommend using an alphabetic mnemonic, or memory guide, favored by doctors: OPQRST.

O = Onset

How did the symptom start?

What were you doing?

Did something you were doing seem to trigger the symptom?

Is it a new symptom or a worsening of an ongoing condition?

P = Provocation or Palliation

What makes the symptom worse (for example, movement, position, breathing, coughing)?

Is there anything that makes the symptom better (rest or medications, for instance)?

Q = Quality

What are the qualities of the symptom?

Do you feel dull or sharp pain?

Does it tingle or burn?

Is it constant or throbbing?

Is there sputum or blood when you cough?

R = Region and Radiation (most relevant for pain)

Where exactly do you feel pain?

Does the pain seem to radiate (spread) to another area?

S = Severity

How severe is the symptom?

How would you rate the pain, with 0 being "no pain" and 10 being "the worst it could be"?

T = Time

How long has the symptom been going on (hours, days, weeks, longer)?

Is the symptom constant, or does it come and go?

A sample symptom tracker is included at the end of this chapter. The tracker will help you ensure that your recollection of your symptoms is accurate. Then, when you do go online, you can keep yourself accountable about whether you *really* feel the symptoms of the condition or disease that you're reading about.

This approach should help to relieve stress when you speak with your doctor about your symptoms. A 2017 study found that when people wrote down their medical history prior to their doctor's visit, 84 percent felt more empowered.[16] Writing down your symptoms and sharing them with your doctor can get your doctor up to speed quickly so that they can focus on working with you to figure out what those symptoms mean.

Moving from an understanding of your symptoms to a diagnosis is a critical step, one that shouldn't be done alone and online without an informed approach. The next chapter will focus on how you can use the internet to look up your symptoms online and make a decision about whether and when to see a doctor.

Symptom Tracker

What is your main symptom?

What is your chief complaint, the thing that is bothering you most?

_____

_____

What is the history of your present illness?

Use the memory trick "OPQRST" to dive into the details.

_____

_____

O = Onset

When did the symptom start?

_____

_____

What were you doing immediately before the onset of the symptom?

_____

_____

Did something you were doing seem to trigger the symptom?

_____

_____

Did the symptom come on all of a sudden or gradually over the course of days or weeks?

_____

_____

If you are having trouble remembering when your symptoms started, consider the last time you felt what you would consider "normal" (your usual state of health). Recall how things changed. What symptom came first? When did the symptom get worse/better?

_____

_____

P = Provocation or Palliation

What makes the symptom worse (movement, position, breathing, coughing, for instance)?

_____

_____

What, if anything, makes the symptom better (for example, rest, medication)?

_____

_____

Q = Quality

What are the qualities of the symptom?

_____

_____

Do you feel dull or sharp pain?

_____

_____

Does it tingle or burn?

_____

_____

Is it constant or throbbing?

_____

_____

Is there sputum or blood when you cough?

_____

_____

Do you have diarrhea? Is the stool watery, loose, or bloody?

_____

_____

R = Region and Radiation (where the pain is felt)

Can you pinpoint the pain with one finger? Or does the pain seem to be more spread out through an area?

_____

_____

Does the pain extend, or radiate, to another area?

_____

_____

S = Severity

How severe is the symptom? How would you rate the pain, with 0 being "no pain" and 10 being "the worst it could be"?

_____

_____

How frequent is the symptom? For example, if you have diarrhea, how many times a day do you have to go?

_____

_____

How much does your symptom interfere with your day-to-day activities? For instance, how often does your cough wake you up from sleep?

_____

_____

T = Time

How long has the symptom been going on (hours, days, weeks, longer)?

_____

_____

Does your symptom come and go? Or has it been constant since the start?

_____

_____

How long does the symptom last?

_____

_____

Do you have short episodes of the symptom, or is it continuous?

_____

_____

Do you have any other related symptoms?

What other symptoms, if any, come with your main symptom? For example, do you have nausea along with your pain? Do you have sweats and/or chills with your fever?

_____

_____

How are you feeling otherwise?

_____

_____

Doctors often ask about other symptoms you have to make sure they have a more complete picture of what you are experiencing. Most doctors ask their patients to complete a review of body systems by filling out a questionnaire that is divided into categories to reflect different parts of the body. Your doctor may decide that one of your other symptoms should be moved up as the main symptom.

You may find it useful to refer to this list to help you accurately note other symptoms. Jot down any symptoms not listed. If any of the symptoms are particularly bothersome, you may find it helpful to use the OPQRST tool above.

SYSTEM	EXAMPLES	
General (constitutional symptoms)	❑ weight loss ❑ excess sweating ❑ fatigue	❑ change in sleeping pattern ❑ change in appetite ❑ fever
Eyes	❑ visual changes ❑ headache ❑ eye pain	❑ double vision ❑ blind spots ❑ floaters
Ears, nose, mouth, and throat (ENT)	❑ runny nose ❑ frequent nosebleeds ❑ sinus pain ❑ stuffy ears ❑ ear pain ❑ vertigo (room spinning)	❑ ringing in ears (tinnitus) ❑ discharge from ears ❑ bleeding gums ❑ toothache ❑ sore throat ❑ pain when swallowing
Heart and circulation (cardiovascular)	❑ chest pain or pressure ❑ shortness of breath with exertion ❑ shortness of breath when lying down ❑ inability to exercise	❑ swelling in the feet ❑ palpitations ❑ faintness or lightheadedness ❑ loss of consciousness ❑ leg cramps
Lungs (respiratory)	❑ cough ❑ sputum ❑ wheeze	❑ coughing up blood ❑ shortness of breath
Gut (gastrointestinal)	❑ abdominal pain ❑ unintentional weight loss ❑ difficulty swallowing ❑ indigestion ❑ bloating ❑ cramping ❑ nausea ❑ heartburn	❑ vomiting ❑ diarrhea ❑ constipation ❑ vomiting blood ❑ blood in stool ❑ smelly, dark, black, tarry stools ❑ change in bowel habits

SYSTEM	EXAMPLES	
Bladder and genitals (genitourinary)	*Urinary* ❑ incontinence ❑ pain with urination ❑ blood in urine ❑ urinating at night ❑ weak stream of urine ❑ delay in starting urination ❑ dribbling *Genital* ❑ discharge ❑ soreness ❑ pain ❑ lumps	*Menstrual* ❑ change in frequency of menses ❑ change in regularity of menses ❑ unusually heavy or light menses ❑ abnormal duration of menses
Muscles and bones (musculoskeletal)	❑ pain ❑ stiffness ❑ joint swelling	❑ decreased range of motion ❑ arthritis
Skin and breast	❑ rash ❑ itching ❑ discoloration ❑ excessive dryness ❑ growth on skin ❑ hair loss ❑ change in nails	Breast ❑ pain ❑ soreness ❑ lumps ❑ discharge
Brain and nerves (nervous)	❑ changes in smell ❑ changes in taste ❑ changes in speech ❑ numbness ❑ tremor	❑ seizures ❑ fainting ❑ headache ❑ pins and needles ❑ poor balance
Psychiatric	❑ depression ❑ change in sleep patterns ❑ anxiety ❑ difficulty concentrating	❑ paranoia ❑ lack of energy ❑ change in personality

SYSTEM	EXAMPLES	
Hormones (endocrine)	❏ increased appetite ❏ increased thirst	❏ increased urine production ❏ intolerance to cold or heat
Blood (hematologic) and lymph (lymphatic)	❏ excess bleeding ❏ easy bruising	❏ swelling of lymph nodes ❏ new lumps or bumps
Allergies (immunologic)	❏ difficulty breathing or throat closing as a result of exposure to anything ❏ hives ❏ runny nose	❏ itchy/watery eyes ❏ allergic response (rash, itch, swelling) to drugs, foods, animals

Please note that the structure of this form is usually constant, but the areas of emphasis can change depending on your doctor's specialty. An eye doctor may list more questions about vision, while a gastrointestinal doctor may have more questions about bowel habits. This form is based on the categories outlined by the Centers for Medicare & Medicaid Services and other online sources.

To learn more about a review of body systems, please see Phillips A, Frank A, Loftin C, Shepherd S. A detailed review of systems: an educational feature. *The Journal for Nurse Practitioners*. 2017;13(10):681–686; Bickley L, Szilagyi PG. *Bates' Guide to Physical Examination and History-Taking*. Philadelphia, PA: Lippincott Williams & Wilkins; 2013.

2 | Moving from Symptoms to a Diagnosis

Erica was a thirty-two-year-old Pilates instructor who prided herself on being in great shape.* When she started feeling pain in her abdomen, she assumed it was a pulled muscle and decided to ease up on her workouts. The pain went away within days. But a few days later, it was back. And this time, it stuck around.

Over the next few weeks, Erica's pain would come and go, seemingly at random. One night, she was reading on her phone when a post on gluten sensitivity caught her eye. The symptoms sounded just like hers. She started to explore. The more she read, the more she was convinced that she had the condition.[1] Erica checked respected websites such as that of the Mayo Clinic. Her symptoms lined up with what she found. The treatment seemed straightforward: a gluten-free diet. She was grateful to take a natural approach and save herself a trip to the doctor.

Erica felt great after the first week of her diet. The pain, nausea, and bloating were gone. And she had more energy than in previous weeks. She raved about the results to her friends, joking that the only weird thing was how her stool had turned black. The color, in fact, was a sign of a life-threatening condition.

---

* Name and personal details have been changed to protect privacy.

Three weeks into her gluten-free diet, Erica awoke and strained just to sit up. Light-headed and weak, she called for her roommate, who took one look at Erica's face and decided she needed to go to the ER. A blur of doctors and a battery of tests later, Erica was given the diagnosis: internal bleeding from an ulcer in her stomach. She'd waited so long after developing the ulcer that she now needed a blood transfusion and an endoscopic procedure to stop the bleeding.

Lying in the hospital bed with an intravenous drip in her arm, Erica wondered how she had landed in her current mess. When she first read the articles on gluten sensitivity, she was sure that was the key to her problems. Abdominal pain was the number one symptom of gluten intolerance. The bloating, the weight loss — all her symptoms lined up. Everything she had read suggested that her symptoms were something that she could manage on her own by changing her diet.

To be perfectly fair, most of us are like Erica. We don't have an innate understanding of what symptoms are suggestive of a critical condition versus those we can manage on our own. And most of us, also like Erica, turn to the internet to help us decide. While some people believe that we should always talk to a doctor if we feel ill, the medical system isn't really set up for that. It can take weeks to get an appointment with a general practitioner, and wait times for ERs are often many hours long. In the end, turning to the internet to figure out whether it's worth going to see a doctor is an understandable move for Erica and for many of us.

What Erica overlooked, though, is the importance of going about her online search in a logical and informed manner. Erica stumbled on the article about gluten sensitivity by accident, and after she read it, every online search she conducted about her symptoms was done in relation to gluten intolerance. Had she looked up her symptoms without any framing around gluten, she would likely have spotted an ulcer as a possible cause, among others, and she may have decided to head to the doctor before things became so severe.

This chapter will give you a set of tools to help you make more informed decisions when you go online to look up symptoms. We'll go over the available scientific evidence and share the techniques doctors use to assess symptoms and come up with a list of possible diagnoses. Using these insights during your online searches will not replace advice from a doctor. However, it may give you a better chance of figuring out the right next step, whether that's going to an ER, booking an appointment with your doctor, or waiting until the symptoms resolve on their own. These insights may also help you communicate more effectively when you do meet with a health care provider.

Think Like Your Doctor: An Approach Based on Clinical Reasoning

Doctors spend years learning how to extract a list of possible diagnoses from a constellation of symptoms and to assess whether symptoms are signs of a critical condition. Yet whenever any one of us sits down in front of a computer to figure out what's wrong, we're essentially attempting to do the same thing, but we're doing it with no training at all. While we obviously can't teach you all the steps a doctor learns to assess symptoms and come to a diagnosis, we can give you insight into their approach, which can improve your own online searches.

The technique we're going to teach you is called *clinical reasoning*. It takes years of training to develop this skill, and it's frankly not reasonable to expect that anyone without proper medical training could learn all the ins and outs of this approach. But we can help you understand the basic idea, which might be valuable to help you make better decisions when browsing for health information online.

Clinical reasoning is, at minimum, a three-step process: (1) acquiring information (data), (2) generating a hypothesis, and (3) recognizing a pattern.[2] Here's how it looks in practice.

A man walks into his doctor's office complaining of shortness of breath. A nurse checks his vital signs. Then the doctor asks the man about his symptoms and medical history and performs a physical examination. This is *data acquisition*: the doctor is trying to find out as much information as possible about the patient and the signs and symptoms he's presenting with.

As the doctor processes the data, she starts formulating some basic ideas around what might be causing her patient's shortness of breath. This is **hypothesis generation**: the doctor starts thinking of the likeliest causes for her patient's difficulty breathing based on her medical knowledge. At this point, in the doctor's mind, the cause might be anything from asthma to heart failure, and it'll take moving to the next step before she's able to narrow it down.

With **pattern recognition**, the doctor matches the patterns of particular conditions and diseases with her patient's signs and symptoms. For doctors, much of this happens automatically. In this case, if the patient's medical history shows that he is a smoker and, along with the difficulty breathing, he is also wheezing and spitting up a lot of phlegm, then the doctor may move chronic obstructive pulmonary disease (COPD) higher up her list of possible causes. If the patient says he's a nonsmoker but he's had fever and chills for a couple of days, the doctor might move lung cancer down the list and pneumonia higher up.

The result of a doctor's clinical reasoning is called a *differential diagnosis*—a short list of possible conditions that the patient might have.[3]

Here's how you can apply clinical reasoning to your own online searches.

Data Acquisition

If you followed the tips in chapter 1, half your data acquisition work is done already. By writing down your symptoms following the OPQRST mnemonic, you captured the first set of data: a detailed breakdown of your symptoms, including when they first started to appear, what you did right before the symptoms occurred, their intensity, and their frequency.

The next step in the data acquisition phase is to pull together your medical history. You want it all in one place, either on paper or electronically. Your medical record should include your current and previous medical issues and surgical procedures, as well as the medical history of close blood relatives. Other factors that affect your health, such as how many alcoholic drinks you have per week, your physical activity, and whether you smoke, should also be included.

At the end of this chapter, we've created a worksheet to help you fill out your medical history. It's good to have this with you when you go online to research your symptoms. On a practical note, it's also useful to take a copy with you whenever you have a doctor's visit. This is especially important if you unexpectedly end up going to an urgent care clinic. In one research study, almost all ER patients surveyed— 99 percent—didn't know the answer to at least one important question about their own medical history.[4] Other research suggests that when a person keeps track of their own medical history, the information is more accurate, and it can be made even more accurate if they track their medical history with the help of their primary care doctor and their doctor's notes.[5,6] Acquiring data during an appointment is time consuming for doctors who don't already know your medical history and of low value for patients since it takes up valuable time. If the data are organized ahead of time in a familiar and useful way, you can get more from your visit and help the doctor focus on more important things, like figuring out what is troubling you.

Hypothesis Generation

When generating a hypothesis, you are essentially coming up with a list of possible conditions that could be causing your symptoms. One question should be driving your thinking at this stage, "What else could it be?"[7] Often, people are looking for a single answer to explain the cause of their symptoms. When we find something that fits, like gluten insensitivity, we stop searching for other possible explanations, which prevents us from finding other possible causes of our symptoms. This phenomenon of drawing a conclusion before all the facts are in is called *cognitive bias*. It has been observed in laypersons and doctors alike.[8] In the latter case, it can lead to missing an important diagnosis. Studies have shown that techniques that reduce or eliminate bias (such as asking, "What else could it be?") can help reduce cognitive bias.[9]

Even before starting an online search, most of us already have a rough guess of what might be causing our problem. It doesn't matter whether we're right or not. What matters is that we write down what we think the problem may be. This initial hypothesis is a useful starting point when we start searching online.

Generally, people begin their online search of health symptoms in one of two places: either a large search engine, such as Yahoo, Bing, or Google, or a trusted health-related website, such as the Mayo Clinic or MedlinePlus (see the box on the following page for tips on how to identify trustworthy websites). If you have no idea what's causing your symptoms, we recommend starting with a large search engine. The reason for this has to do with what's happening on the back end of the search engine. The technologies that underlie many current search engines—including natural language processing, machine learning, and a knowledge graph—help return better results than a single website can generally provide.

If you were to search "neck pain all day, worse with movement," that search is broken down by Google into its various entities: "neck pain," "movement," and "day." The search engine then uses some combination of machine learning, natural language processing, and the knowledge graph—essentially a vast database of hundreds of millions of separate entities such as places, people, movies, foods—to return a list of websites that reference all three separate entities, prioritized to some degree based on which web page might be most relevant to you.[10]

This is a simplified take on what's going on, but here's why it matters to you: when you go online to search your symptoms, you should focus on your key symptoms and perhaps one or two of its most significant traits. Since shorter queries generally work better than longer queries, you want to focus your initial search on the main symptom (perhaps pain, dizziness, or nausea) and its key traits, which could be location (where on the body it hurts), duration (acute or chronic), or any other associated symptoms that accompany the main one (maybe neck pain or fever).

If you're taking medications for another condition, you'll want to try at least one search where you include the name of your medications along with your symptoms. This will help you determine whether your symptoms are a side effect of one of your current medications.

Trustworthy Websites

When you've done a search on the internet and are reading through your search results, it's important to recognize which sites are reliable and which ones aren't.[1] Generally speaking, government websites are quite reliable. These are easy to spot since all government sites in the United States have ".gov" at the end of the URL. So, when you see online health information presented by the National Library of Medicine (https://www.medlineplus.gov/), for example, you know it's going to have reliable content. The National Health Service, which is run by the UK government, has a detailed website (https://www.nhs.uk/) that is a trustworthy resource. Other reliable sources of information are academic institutions, such as Harvard University or Johns Hopkins University. These sites generally have ".edu" at the end of the URL, although some like the Mayo Clinic might have ".org" (https://www.mayoclinic.org/).

Many nonprofit sites are also quite useful. These sites may represent professional bodies that have a significant amount of information about single conditions or diseases, such as the site of the

---

American Diabetes Association (https://www.diabetes.org/). These sites often have ".org" in the URL. That said, some nonprofit organizations were created to promote a specific viewpoint and may be biased. For example, with Lyme disease, there are two conflicting views: one side sees the disease as treatable by a short course of antibiotics, while the other suggests that Lyme disease is a chronic condition that requires long-term treatment. Each viewpoint is supported by powerful nonprofit organizations, each with their own ".org" website and each driving their own interpretation of the facts. Additional research is required before deciding to use a nonprofit organization as your main source of information. This leads to another piece of advice—try to confirm what you find by looking at multiple credible sources. This makes it more likely that you will find information that is accurate.

One thing to keep in mind with authoritative websites affiliated with governments, academic institutions, and nonprofits is liability. There are legal implications for those institutions if their website provides reassurance to a user and the symptom turns out to be a serious condition. These websites generally encourage users to speak with a medical provider as a way to protect themselves from any legal action.

Nonauthoritative websites, such as blogs, Facebook, and other types of forums, are also useful but for different reasons. They often include personal posts, written in everyday language. While not necessarily backed by science or research, the stories on these sites may play a role in making health information more accessible and relatable. For example, if someone decided to take an over-the-counter treatment for a muscle injury, they may find useful information on these sites about how long it generally takes for the treatment to work.

It is also important to remember that these nonauthoritative websites may give a skewed picture based on one person's experience. If someone gets a red, pimply rash and it resolves on its own, they move on with their lives and forget about it. However, if this red, pimply rash turns out to be a rare sign of cancer, then they may be prompted to write about it in a blog, post it on social media, or share it with a local news outlet. The result is that an online search for "red pimply rash" may suggest that it is a sign of cancer even though, in the majority of cases, it is not serious and resolves on its own. Any information from a nonauthoritative source needs to be double-checked with a more authoritative source.

Some websites offer symptom checkers as an easy way for a person to quickly diagnose themselves based on their set of symptoms. The checkers generally ask users a series of questions to get more information about risk factors and symptoms. Then, they map this to a series of possible diagnoses to come up with matches and some recommendations. There are several downsides to the currently available trackers. First, there are serious concerns about accuracy. A study in *BMJ* looked at twenty-three different symptom checkers and found that the correct diagnosis was listed first in only 34 percent of cases.[2] Further, the advice regarding the urgency of a person's condition was incorrect anywhere from 22 percent to 67 percent of the time. The main issue was that the checker would recommend that users seek medical attention when self-care may have been sufficient, suggesting that symptom checkers are overly risk averse. Given this study, and others like it,[3] it is probably wise for you to do additional research on any results that come from a symptom checker.

The bottom line is that all these types of online resources can be very useful if you understand their strengths and weaknesses. It is important not to rely on any one of them exclusively, but rather to use a combination of sources.

Reading your online search results is the most challenging part of hypothesis generation. It's important not to panic if a rare and scary condition appears in your results and enters your list of possible conditions. There's a saying among doctors that is useful for you to keep in mind when you feel yourself start to panic: When you hear hoofbeats, think horses not zebras. Rare conditions are exactly that—rare. There are other conditions that are more common but equally scary, like cancer and heart disease. Don't panic and assume that one of these conditions is causing your symptoms, but don't ignore it either. The goal here is to think of all possible causes ("What else could it be?"). The next stage, pattern recognition, is where we take the broad list and start narrowing it down.

Pattern Recognition

For doctors, matching a set of symptoms against a possible disease or condition is an almost automatic process thanks to their years of training and experience. For you, pattern recognition will be slower and more methodical, but you'll follow a similar approach.

Armed with your medical history and a description of your symptoms, start going through the list of possible conditions generated by your initial online search. For each one, you're looking for specifics that match your symptoms and are in line with your medical history. Group your conditions into three possible categories: Very Likely, Somewhat Likely, and Unlikely. Here's where a website like WebMD or MedlinePlus may prove useful—when you're exploring a specific condition, looking for a description of how that condition presents itself, and seeing if it matches your pattern of symptoms.

If your main symptom is fatigue, you might start by looking up "possible causes of fatigue." If anemia is on the list, and if you've had it before, you might explore anemia in a bit more detail. Is anemia an ongoing part of your medical history, or did it occur only once for a very specific reason? Do other symptoms of anemia match up with yours? If so, you might want to put anemia in the Very Likely column. If anemia has never been a problem for you and you are not at risk, you might put it in the Unlikely category. As more of your symptoms and history match a description of a given condition, the more likely it is that the condition is your possible diagnosis. If very few items match, and it is a stretch to match your progression of symptoms to the description of how the disease typically presents, it is probably fine to take the condition off your list.

There is an interesting study that gives insight into how people conduct their online health searches.[11] The researchers noticed a pattern in which a person would skim a website about a condition and then move on to another condition. They called this type of searcher the *flounderer*. Generally speaking, flounderers would do better to go into a little more depth on each site. Another tactic that some people in the study used was to open separate tabs to get definitions of words they didn't understand. This is a handy way to understand unfamiliar terms without losing track of the main article.

Late night television host Jimmy Kimmel once told a story about pattern recognition in action. He'd noticed a sharp pain on one side of his body, near the belt region. A self-confessed hypochondriac, he immediately went online to research his symptoms. Appendicitis was one possible cause. When he looked up the details of the condition, he was surprised to see just how well his symptoms matched up. The location of the pain was correct, he was also suffering from bouts of nausea, and he was within the common age range affected. According to the story Jimmy told, "I diagnosed myself. I called my doctor and I told him my appendix was about to burst, and he laughed at me. And then I went in and he said, 'Congratulations, you're the first person who's ever correctly diagnosed himself on the internet!'"

There are a number of other resources, aside from the internet, to help you determine what could be causing your symptoms. Some medical centers and health insurance providers offer virtual urgent care, so you can schedule an online consultation with a certified health care provider who can answer questions you may have about your symptoms and give you more direction on whether you should seek help immediately or wait. See the box on the following page for a list of other resources that may be available to you. You can also search online to see what services are in your area.

Other Places to Turn beyond the Internet

Many people may not be aware of other options available to them beyond turning to the internet, visiting their doctor, or going to the ER. Below is a list of other options that may be available to you. All these options can help you make a more informed decision about whether you have a true emergency or something that can be handled in a less urgent setting.

Nurse Triage Phone Lines

Well before the origin of the internet, nurse triage phone lines were a main source of support for people feeling ill and wondering what to do. The service, which is often provided by a doctor's office or health insurance company, connects people to a trained nurse over the phone. The nurse will go through a series of questions with you to determine whether your symptoms warrant a visit to the ER. If the symptoms don't warrant a visit, the nurse will recommend treatments to try at home and then will check back in to see if your condition has improved. It is good practice to ask your doctor's office and your health insurance provider whether they have nurse triage lines and to keep these numbers handy in case of any unexpected health-related event.

Poison Control Line

A specialized type of phone triage is the one that is offered by poison control. Here, a poison expert will assess the situation and help figure out next steps. The poison control line can offer support if you or someone you know has swallowed something that may be harmful. A poison control line can also be helpful if you fear that you may have inhaled or rubbed up against a harmful substance or even if a substance may have gotten in your eye. In the United States, you can text "poison" to 484848 to find your local poison control hotline, or visit the National Capital Poison Center website (https://www.poison.org/).

Virtual Appointments

Aside from triage phone lines, advances in technology have created a number of easy ways to reach health care providers without going to a clinic. Some medical centers and health insurance providers offer virtual urgent care appointments, which are a good option in situations where you are not sure if your symptoms are severe enough to warrant an urgent care visit or not. A telemedicine provider can walk through your symptoms and help you come up with a plan. Since they cannot do a physical examination, it is possible that you may still need to go to a facility to be seen in person, though in many cases the telemedicine consult is sufficient. Indeed, Kaiser Permanente found that digital interactions topped in-person visits in 2017.[1]

There are also online forums such as HealthTap, telemedicine offerings such as Amwell, Doctor on Demand, and Teladoc, and text messaging–based services such as Lemonaid Health. Online forums offer the least amount of support and are often public. Here, a health care provider, forum participant, or both answer questions posed by a user. By design, there is a rather limited amount of context provided to those answering the question. These forums are best suited to address a focused question that isn't particularly urgent.

Pharmacies and Other Urgent Care Centers

As the number of online solutions has multiplied, so has the number of in-person options. In response to the overuse of ERs, urgent care centers have cropped up across the United States. Pharmacy companies such as CVS and Walgreens to retailers like Walmart now have clinics inside stores to manage urgent conditions as well as nonurgent issues like vaccinations. These are called retail clinics. The pharmacists themselves may also be a useful resource.

Knowing When It's Time to Act: Clinical Reasoning in Practice

But what happens when you're not 100 percent sure whether your symptoms match a condition? Do you wait it out at home and hope for the best, or do you head straight to the ER if there's a condition on your Somewhat Likely list that you're concerned about?

Doug Hennig is the chief technology officer and vice president of a software company in Canada. In early 2012, Doug was living in Saskatchewan, where temperatures regularly hover below thirty-two degrees Fahrenheit (zero degrees Celsius) during the winter months. A few months into the new year, he was taking out the garbage and slipped on an icy sidewalk. He could still walk, albeit with a limp, so he assumed it was just a sprained ankle. His wife, Peggy, wasn't so sure. She insisted that he go to a walk-in clinic for an X-ray and, sure enough, he had a double break in his fibula that needed surgery. Peggy's instincts had been right—Doug had needed to see a doctor because of his fall.

Fast-forward two weeks post-surgery, and Doug was feeling virtually no pain. His son was competing in a speed skating championship in Winnipeg, in the neighboring province. Since he was feeling better, Doug and his wife decided to drive the five hours to watch their son compete. Shortly after dinner on the first day of the competition, Doug started to feel a bit feverish. "We were going up and down the stairs in the bleachers, and it was cold inside the rink, as you'd expect," Doug said in a conversation in late 2019. "I felt like I had a little bit of a fever, and my back was a little bit sore. But I just put it down to me overexerting myself while I should have been recovering from the broken ankle."

But then, the next night, Doug woke up in excruciating pain. "It felt like somebody stabbed me with a knife in the ribs. It was the most painful thing. Every breath felt like someone was stabbing me again with a knife," he said. "So I got up and took some muscle relaxants, propped some pillows behind myself and after they kicked in, I was able to fall asleep sitting up."

The next day, as he and Peggy were driving back to their hometown, they talked about what they thought was causing the pain. They were essentially shifting into hypothesis generation in the clinical reasoning process, while keeping Doug's recent medical surgery and list of symptoms in mind. Doug still had a fever, but the rib pain and back pain had become more manageable. "When we got home, I sat down on the couch, took out the iPad, and started Googling 'fever after surgery' because we figured it was maybe related to the problem with my ankle, though we didn't know for sure." Doug came across a few websites that suggested that fever after surgery was most commonly associated with a post-surgery infection.

Here's where Doug started moving into pattern recognition, trying to match his specific set of symptoms with the possible causes of his fever and pain. With a post-surgery infection, there's normally pain and redness in the area where the surgery took place. Doug didn't have any pain or redness near his ankle, so he doubted an infection was the cause. He moved this condition into the Unlikely column.

A few other causes also came up, including fever caused by post-operative drugs and an infection of a major organ, but none of those seemed like a fit for what Doug was feeling. Those causes went into the Unlikely column as well. As he read through his online results, one thing did seem possible: a pulmonary embolism, which occurs when a blood clot forms—like in a leg that's been recently immobilized—and travels to the lungs. But pulmonary embolisms often come with shortness of breath, which Doug hadn't experienced, and they aren't particularly common, so Doug considered this Unlikely.

"I was reading the description of a pulmonary embolism to my wife, and I mentioned to her that it was fatal if untreated. She immediately said, 'Let's go to the ER tomorrow and just get this checked out because it may not be that, but if it's fatal if untreated then that seems like a serious consequence for not getting it checked out.' I agreed, though I was sure that it was not it. But maybe if I go to the ER," thought Doug, "they'll be able to figure out what it is."

When Doug and his wife arrived at the ER, the doctors moved fast because Peggy had told the triage nurse about Doug's recent medical history and ankle surgery. The ER doctor suggested that the fever and pain were caused by either a clot or pneumonia, and he suggested some tests to narrow down the diagnosis. An X-ray and a CT scan later, they had it. Doug had both pneumonia and a pulmonary embolism. The pneumonia was neither severe nor life-threatening, but the embolism was. Fortunately, since Doug and his wife had gone to the ER early and the clot was small, the treatment was straightforward and relatively quick: blood thinners for the next six months.[12]

Doug's approach is the one we want you to take as well. Use clinical reasoning to narrow down the list of possible conditions causing your symptoms, then consider the following suggestions to determine what to do next:

- If one of the conditions on your list is potentially fatal or could lead to permanent or severe damage, get yourself checked out immediately. Oftentimes, a website will list *red flag symptoms*. If *any* of these symptoms match up with what you're feeling, you should see a doctor.

- If many of your symptoms match those of a life-threatening condition, but there's one major red flag symptom missing—such as a rash or high fever that you haven't yet experienced—consider using another resource, like a nurse triage phone line, to help you make the decision about seeing a doctor (see the box on pages 32–33). If you feel comfortable waiting, be sure you understand what signs to look for that indicate worsening of your condition, and be prepared to seek help if needed.

- If a serious condition is on your Somewhat Likely or Very Likely list of conditions but isn't immediately life-threatening (something like cancer), consider booking an appointment with your regular doctor instead of seeking emergency care. While it can be hard to resist the urge to get tested immediately, ERs are set up to deal with emergencies. If there is no immediate, life-threatening emergency, chances are the ER doctors will ultimately refer you to your primary care doctor, but only after charging you for the visit. Assuming that the condition you fear you may have isn't immediately life-threatening, it's generally better to go directly to primary care in the first place.

These are intended only as suggestions to help provide some guidance. If you think that a condition is serious, you should meet with your doctor to discuss your symptoms and the possible conditions that could be causing them. Making the most out of that visit is what we turn to next.

Your Medical History

Medical Conditions

List all your current medical conditions and the year in which you were diagnosed:

_____

_____

_____

List any medical conditions that have resolved:

_____

_____

_____

Sometimes, if you're struggling with many conditions, it's hard to remember them all or the ones that you were diagnosed with in the past. Here is a short checklist to help jog your memory and make sure you have a complete list.

Cancer	Multiple Sclerosis
Heart Attack	Stroke/TIA
Heart Murmur	ADHD
High Blood Pressure	Alcohol Abuse
High Cholesterol	Anorexia/Bulimia
Diabetes	Anxiety Disorder
Pneumonia	Drug Dependency
Asthma	Depression
COPD	HIV/AIDS
Broken Bones	Chlamydia or Gonorrhea
Concussion	Genital Herpes
Seizure	Thyroid Disease
Migraine	Chronic Kidney Disease

Kidney Stones

Glaucoma

Cataracts

Anemia

Bleeding Disorder

Blood Clot/Clotting Disorder

Polycystic Ovary Syndrome

Hearing Loss

Hay Fever

Eczema

Recurrent Sinus Infections

Celiac Disease

Irritable Bowel Syndrome

Stomach Ulcer

Ulcerative Colitis or
    Crohn's Disease

Polyps in Colon

Arthritis

Surgeries

List your prior surgeries:

_____

_____

_____

It can be hard to remember surgeries if they took place a long time ago. Here is a short checklist to jog your memory and make sure you have a complete list.

O (Date: _____) Appendectomy

O (Date: _____) Adenoidectomy

O (Date: _____) Ear Tubes

O (Date: _____) Gallbladder Removal

O (Date: _____) Knee ACL Repair (Left/Right)

O (Date: _____) Knee Arthroscopy (Left/Right)

O (Date: _____) Ovarian Cyst Removal

O (Date: _____) Tonsillectomy

O (Date: _____) Weight Loss Surgery

O (Date: _____) Other Prior Surgeries

Medications

List all medications that you are currently taking, including the dosage and start date. It might be helpful to note if you need refills as a reminder for your next visit. Also list any supplements, herbs, and natural health products and over-the-counter medications that you take.

List your current medications, including over-the-counter ones:

_____

_____

_____

List any supplements, herbs, and natural health products:

_____

_____

_____

Are you allergic to any medications? If yes, which ones?

_____

_____

_____

Family Medical History

A standard family medical history usually lists major diseases of your closest blood relatives. We developed a chart you can use to begin tracking your family history below. We encourage you to adapt this list as needed, in conversation with your doctor. The US government has also created an online tool to collect your family history (https://phgkb.cdc.gov/FHH/html/index.html), which you may find useful.

DOES YOUR IMMEDIATE FAMILY HAVE ANY OF THE FOLLOWING?				
	Mother	Father	Siblings	Grandparents
Alcoholism				
Blood Clots/Clotting Disorders				
Cancer: Breast				
Cancer: Colon				
Cancer: Melanoma				
Cancer: Other				
Diabetes				
Drug Dependency				
Heart Disease				
High Blood Pressure				
High Cholesterol				
Mental Illness				

Searching *for* Health

List any significant family history in your first-degree relatives:

Biological mother:

_____

_____

Biological father:

_____

_____

Siblings:

_____

_____

List any significant family history in your second-degree relatives (uncles/aunts, grandparents):

_____

_____

Women's Health History

Date of last menstrual cycle: _____

Age at first menstruation: _____

Age at menopause: _____

Total number of pregnancies: _____

Number of live births: _____

Pregnancy complications: _____

Last pap smear: _____

Sexual History

Many studies show that people are reluctant to bring up their sexual health with a health care professional. Writing down questions as well as details of symptoms can help.

Are you sexually active? If yes, with men or women? Or with both?

_____

How many active partners do you have?

_____

Do you use contraception? If yes, what kind?

_____

Do you have any sexual issues to discuss?

_____

Social History

Many doctors will ask about your history of alcohol, tobacco, and drug use. Although not every doctor asks about these, it's useful to include this information, as well as any relevant information about recent travel, your home environment, and your occupational environment.

Do you smoke tobacco? If yes, how many cigarettes per day?

_____

Do you use e-cigarettes? If yes, how many times per day?

_____

Do you drink alcohol? If yes, how many drinks per week?

_____

Do you drink caffeinated beverages? If yes, what type
(coffee/tea/soda), and how many per day?

_____

Do you use recreational drugs? If yes, what type and how often?

_____

Do you exercise? How many minutes per week on average?

_____

Do you get enough sleep? Do you feel rested when you wake up?

_____

Who else lives in the home with you?

_____

What kind of work do you do?

_____

Have you traveled in the last year? If yes, where?

_____

Is there any relationship between your experiences at work, travel, or
home and the symptoms you have?

_____

What is your highest education level?

_____

3 | Meeting with Your Doctor about Your Diagnosis

Dr. B had been looking forward to her patient Martin's appointment for a while. Martin had been diagnosed with type 2 diabetes five years earlier, and Dr. B was concerned about how he was managing his condition. He'd missed a number of recent appointments, and she had just learned that he had been hospitalized because of an abscess that could have been avoided if he'd been controlling his diabetes better.

In Dr. B's mind, today was a prime opportunity to seriously talk to Martin about what was going to happen if he didn't control his diabetes. It was also probably the only time she'd get a chance to confirm that Martin knew how to treat his abscess so it wouldn't get worse and to make sure that he was packing his wound, a term used to describe filling an open wound with wet gauze or other packing material to prevent infection and help the wound heal.

Martin was eager to meet with Dr. B as well. The pain around his abscess was so excruciating he couldn't even change the bandages. On top of that, he'd been feeling dizzy, and his vision had started to blur. He was really beginning to worry about what was happening to his body.

As Martin waited in Dr. B's examination room, he went over the things he wanted to get out of the appointment: a reason for why he was feeling dizzy, a reason for his blurry vision, and some kind of advice or support to help him manage his pain. When Dr. B walked in, the first thing she asked Martin was how he was doing. "Better than last week," he replied, trying to be positive.

"Better than last week?" asked Dr. B. "I heard you were in the hospital. Is the nurse coming every single day for the dressing change?" Within the first minute, Dr. B was onto one of her two agenda items—teaching Martin to pack his wound—and Martin had no time to raise any of his other concerns.

The medical community became aware of Martin's appointment with Dr. B when it was written up in the *Journal of Clinical Outcomes Management* because of how poor the communication was between Martin and his doctor.[1] Dr. B was focused almost entirely on wound care, whereas Martin was more concerned about his pain and what his dizziness and blurred vision could mean. The authors give a verbatim account of what took place after the initial rough start between Dr. B and Martin:

> *After the patient reveals he no longer has any packing in the wound because "it just hurt too bad" to replace (an elaboration on his agenda of Pain), he introduces his second agenda, Blurry Eyes.*
>
> > Patient: *I got my new glasses . . . But my eyes are still real blurry. The test results . . . they told me I don't have any glaucoma.*
>
> *The patient offers test results to corroborate the importance of his second agenda, but after a lengthy search the physician finds that the papers discuss a 2-year-old colonoscopy for hemorrhoids. The physician then attempts to switch the agenda back to Wound Care.*

This scenario plays out in doctors' offices in different variations every single day. Both doctors and patients, knowingly or not, have their own agenda when walking into any appointment. Because of how rushed most appointments are, the patient and doctor often end up talking over each other in an effort to get to all their points. Yet the research shows that this approach isn't good for either the patient or the doctor.

A National Academy of Medicine report from 2015 highlights the importance of communication between the patient and doctor to improve diagnosis.[2] This chapter will help you make the most of your time at the doctor's office and give you the tools to communicate effectively and raise your concerns in a way that your doctor, or any doctor, will be able to understand and take into consideration. It summarizes some of the most effective approaches mentioned in the literature, such as preparing ahead of time, asking questions, and making sure you understand what your doctor has said.[3,4] We've also included some suggested scripts at the end of the chapter, which are useful tools to encourage you to bring up important health information and help guide conversations with your doctor.[5]

Think Like Your Doctor: Before the Appointment

Write Down Your Agenda

Think about what you want to get out of your appointment. Do you want to feel better? Are you looking to get a better understanding of your disease? Change your medications? Before you meet with your doctor, write your agenda items down so you can refer to them during your appointment. Most doctors have an agenda that is some combination of learning about new symptoms, looking for clues in a physical examination, ordering tests and treatments, and monitoring chronic conditions. You want to be sure that your agenda isn't lost or consumed by your doctor's.

To help you as you think through how you'll craft your agenda, we've included a worksheet at the end of the chapter. It will help you make sure that you're not forgetting anything as you list your agenda items. An agenda will also help you prioritize your issues so that you can make sure the most important items are addressed.

Book Your Appointment Appropriately

If your agenda is long or there are a few major items you know you'll want to discuss in detail, let the office know this when you call to book your appointment. Some doctors' offices allow you to book back-to-back appointments or have extra time for longer visits. Not every doctor offers this, and not every insurance plan will pay for extended visits, but it never hurts to ask.

Even if your doctor doesn't offer longer appointments, it's worth asking the person booking your appointment if there are other options available. They might be able to schedule you for two appointments within a week so that you have additional time reserved if you need it. They may also be able to give you a sense of when the office is busy and when things slow down, so you can book an appointment when it's likely that your doctor won't be as rushed. You may even be able to email your agenda items to the doctor ahead of the visit so they come into the meeting prepared.

If no options are offered, try at the very least to book your appointment early in the morning when there is a much higher chance that your appointment will start on time. The harsh reality is that doctors rarely have extra time, and it will take some effort on your part to go against the grain and be heard.

Help with Data Gathering

As mentioned in previous chapters, data gathering can be a time-consuming process for doctors. If you can do some of the work in advance, you and your doctor can focus on more important topics during your appointment. If you followed the tips in chapters 1 and 2, then all you need to do is make sure to have your symptom tracker and your medical history filled out and with you during your meeting.

Most clinics and medical providers now give you the opportunity to fill out a medical history prior to meeting with your provider. If you have this opportunity, take advantage of it and fill out the questionnaire at home before you go. If your provider doesn't offer this, make sure to show up at least fifteen to twenty minutes in advance of your appointment and ask the staff at reception whether you can submit your information before your meeting.

Sometimes, insurance companies require a doctor to go through your medical history in person as part of the visit to show that a complete history was taken and justify payment for the doctor's time. In this case, have your medical history and symptom tracker with you in the examination room to refer to or to share directly with your provider. This can make the data gathering portion of the visit much more efficient.

Think Like Your Doctor: During the Appointment

Raise Your Agenda Early

Once you walk into your appointment, your doctor will likely give you the opportunity to introduce your agenda, with a friendly "So what brings you in today?" If your doctor doesn't ask a question like this, don't be shy about bringing it up yourself early in the conversation. If your doctor immediately starts in on their agenda and doesn't give you time to speak, it's fine to respond with something like, "I'm looking forward to discussing the items you want to talk about during today's visit, but I also want to let you know a couple things I wanted to address too, so we can be sure we have time for it all today." This acknowledges the doctor's agenda but reminds them that you also have things you want to talk about.

Why bring up your agenda early in the conversation? Most doctors have an agenda and a structure in mind for each visit. If you let them know your agenda early in the conversation, it gives the doctor the opportunity to tailor the visit to make time for the items on both of your agendas. Several research studies show that having an agenda and proactively bringing it up early in the conversation can improve your visit.[6]

If you don't bring your agenda up early in the appointment, it can sometimes cause unnecessary friction. Doctors often talk about something called the *doorknob phenomenon*. This occurs when the appointment is over and the doctor is reaching for the door, but the patient says what are often dreaded words, "Oh, by the way. . . ." At best, the rest of that sentence is a quick comment about an easily dismissed complaint. At worst, it's the start of a whole new conversation about a symptom or concern that should have been addressed much earlier.

If there were unlimited time for every appointment, this wouldn't be an issue. But with doctors increasingly pressured to keep their appointments to time, raising a major concern at the end of your appointment may leave you without enough time to have an in-depth conversation about an issue you care about.

Bring your agenda items up early, then let your doctor do their job and guide the next steps about what to talk about and when. Since your doctor knows what you're concerned about, they'll almost always return to these points later in the appointment. Before the end of your visit, take one last look at your agenda and remind your doctor of any lingering concerns, with the understanding that you may need a follow-up visit if there isn't enough time.

Gather New Data

Bring a pen and paper to your appointment, and take notes during your visit. Authorities such as the Agency for Healthcare Research and Quality encourage note-taking as a way of remembering what was said.[7,8] One study on patient recall showed that patients only remembered half of the important points raised by their doctors during their appointments.[9] You don't need to take notes throughout the entire appointment, but if the doctor says something you want to look up later or mentions a medication, test, next step, or diagnosis, you may want to stop the conversation and take a moment to write it down.

In addition to note-taking being helpful for remembering key points, it also slows down the pace of the conversation. We talk at about 110 to 150 words per minute but write at fifteen to thirty-five words per minute. Slowing the momentum of the conversation will give you more time to process critical pieces of information.

Some people may prefer to record their meeting. Studies show that people who have access to recordings of their appointments are more satisfied and feel a greater understanding of the issues than those who don't.[10] While some doctors are fine with this, and some medical centers actually encourage it, many providers may be uncomfortable with how the recording might be shared, especially in today's social media climate. If you would like to record your conversation, ask your doctor if it's okay. If your doctor isn't comfortable with being recorded, be respectful of their choice,[11] and ask them to help you write down and remember important information after the meeting.

Get a Sense of the Working Diagnosis and Plan

If your appointment was to discuss symptoms of concern, you can expect that at the end of the conversation your doctor is forming a working diagnosis and plan. The working diagnosis is their best guess of what they think is going on. The plan is what they want to do next.

Most providers will share a simplified version of these thoughts with you. If they don't talk about what they think is going on and instead jump directly to ordering tests, you should feel comfortable politely stepping in and asking your doctor to explain their working diagnosis.

In some cases, a clinical diagnosis can be made without tests, based solely on a person's history and a physical examination. For example, a hernia is usually a clinical diagnosis: a person complains of a lump or swelling, and the hernia is confirmed during the physical examination.

In other cases, tests will be necessary, but the doctor will still have a working diagnosis that they are using to guide their thinking.

In addition to a working or clinical diagnosis, your doctor is probably also forming a differential diagnosis. A differential diagnosis is a list of other possible, but less likely, conditions that a person might have. It's the difference between "It seems like sunburn" (working diagnosis) and "It seems like sunburn, but there's a very unlikely chance that it could also be lupus or dermatomyositis" (differential diagnosis).

Generally speaking, it's worth asking your doctor what their differential diagnosis is. If they don't offer it first themselves, consider asking your doctor the same thing you asked yourself when you were looking up your symptoms online, "What else could it be?" This will give you a sense of their differential diagnosis. If you have done your own online research, see if the conditions you were considering as likely or possible causes of your symptoms are on your doctor's list. If they aren't, consider asking why not.

Another question to consider asking is "Do all my symptoms fit the diagnosis?" This will give you a sense of how well the diagnosis explains your symptoms. If all the symptoms do not fit, it might be worth asking if the doctor thinks there is more than one thing going on. You may also want to go online after the visit and explore the other conditions that the doctor is considering further.

That said, we recognize that it can be anxiety-inducing to delve too deeply into the differential diagnosis. The differential diagnosis may include rare but serious conditions that could lead to unnecessary stress and anxiety if you dwell on the possibilities for too long. Some people prefer to cross that bridge when they come to it. In other words, if the diagnosis is confirmed, they will deal with it at that point. Others prefer to be more informed about each step along the way. It may be helpful to reflect on where you stand and then ask questions accordingly.

Repeat What You Hear

To keep things in perspective during your appointment and reduce the risk of misunderstanding, we recommend that you repeat back what your doctor says to you about the diagnosis. A doctor may rattle off a long list of possible diagnoses and tests, which can be confusing. Repeating the information back helps eliminate some of that confusion.

For example, a doctor may say, "I think your chest discomfort and nausea might be gastritis, so I'm ordering a test for a bacterium called *H. pylori*. If this comes back positive, you'll need antibiotics. But I'm also going to run some tests now to rule out the possibility of a cardiac problem." If a patient replies with, "So, if I understand correctly, you think it's gastritis, so you're testing for that, but it could also be a heart attack?" then the doctor knows the patient fully understands what could be causing their symptoms. However, if a patient replies with, "So, if I understand correctly, you're doing tests because you think it could be a heart attack?" then the doctor has a chance to remind the patient that the most likely cause of their symptoms is probably something less harmful—gastritis. By repeating back what you hear, your doctor can clear up any confusion and help you put your worst fears and anxieties to rest.

This exact method is taught to health care providers, particularly nurses, and is called *teach-back*.[12] The Institute for Healthcare Improvement explains teach-back in a way most of us can relate to: "The last time you ordered take-out, did the restaurant staff read your order back to you to make sure it was right? Read-back is a simple way to close the loop on a communication, ensuring that both parties share the same information. Teach-back is a similar technique that providers can use with patients to ensure they've effectively communicated their health advice or information."

Express Concerns

As the visit starts to wind down, be sure to express any lingering questions. Are there things you didn't understand? Anything you're not comfortable with? Look at your agenda, and see if there's anything that was not covered.

We recognize that it's not always easy to raise concerns with your doctor. Your health care provider probably knows it too. Within the medical community, the hesitation people feel about raising questions is often called *white coat silence*.[13] Research suggests that people hesitate to bring up information because they worry about the doctor's reaction or are afraid of being embarrassed or labelled as difficult. It can be particularly challenging to raise questions about information that you found online. Some doctors are receptive to patients who have done their own online research, but some are not.[14,15] It's perhaps because of this reason that some people choose to disguise the fact that they found health information online.[16]

The Power Dynamic in the Exam Room

It's important to recognize the imbalance of power that often exists in the doctor's office. Doctors have undergone years of training to get to their current position and, as a rule, people accept that doctors are deserving of respect and consideration. Unfortunately, though it is rare, there are cases when doctors take advantage of the power dynamic and violate their patients' trust.

There are steps you can take if you feel uncomfortable during a doctor's appointment or physical examination. You can ask your doctor to stop the exam at any time. You can ask for a nurse or other chaperone from the clinic to be present for your physical exam or during your entire appointment. You can also invite a friend or family member to come into the doctor's office with you and stay during your exam.

Sexual abuse by a health care provider is a serious violation of medical ethics and the law. If you think you have experienced sexual abuse by a medical professional, report it. Contact the hospital, doctor's office, or facility where you experienced the abuse and report the behavior. Contact your local law enforcement as well or any other authority in your community who can step in to prevent the situation from happening again. Consider filing a report with the state medical board, which issues physician licenses. It can be hard to speak up about abuse by a health care provider, but doing so will help prevent the same abuse from happening to others.

The way you bring up issues or online information with your doctor will depend on your relationship with them, but we encourage you to be honest and open. One way to frame it is to explain that you are engaged in your health and have certain concerns. In general, doctors are happiest when patients are engaged. If your doctor isn't, you may want to seek a second opinion to help you feel more comfortable and confident with the decisions you're making.

Figure Out What's Next

Most doctors will order tests to confirm their working or clinical diagnosis and to rule out the conditions that make up their differential diagnosis. While testing is important, it's hard for the average person to fully understand which tests are necessary and which are not. Some doctors do order too many tests in an attempt to be thorough, or they don't order the right test and they miss the diagnosis. At the same time, patients often ask for tests that they don't need. Not only is overtesting costly—to insurers, the government, and the patients themselves as premiums and copays rise—but tests can also have negative side effects or trigger additional procedures that are also unnecessary.[17]

All that said, testing is important, and the solution isn't to automatically say no to more tests. The goal is to make sure that you have the right test at the right time. Generally speaking, we recommend that you trust the tests that your doctor orders. We also want you to make sure that you understand why tests are being done and what conditions the test will help either rule out or confirm.

The American Board of Internal Medicine Foundation has created a campaign called Choosing Wisely to help people understand their testing options (https://www.choosingwisely.org/). They recommend that people ask their doctor five basic questions:

1. Do I really need this test or procedure?

2. What are the risks and side effects?

3. Are there simpler, safer options?

4. What happens if I don't do anything?

5. How much does it cost?

Your doctor should be able to give you comprehensive answers to the first four questions. The last question on costs may not be as easy for your doctor to answer. Often, with medical tests, there is an amount that your doctor's office will charge, an amount that your insurance company will pay, and a smaller amount that you as the patient will pay. If you don't have insurance and are paying for a test out of pocket, then your doctor's office may charge a different rate than what they charge the insurance companies.

NPR and Kaiser Health News help people investigate their medical bills and cases of being overcharged. In one extreme case, a woman was prescribed painkillers following back surgery.[18] During a follow-up visit, staff at the clinic asked her to leave a urine sample, which she thought was routine. A year later, the lab sent her a bill for $17,850 for testing for a variety of drugs, including cocaine, methadone, anti-anxiety medication, and several other drugs she had never heard of.

While that kind of price gouging isn't the norm, almost all of us have been surprised by the unexpected costs of testing. There are a few tips that may help you save money on testing or, at the very least, give you a better sense of how much your tests will cost:

- Ask your doctor's office for the exact name of the test requested. If possible, get the CPT codes of the tests that have been ordered.[19]

- Call your health insurance company to ask if the test is covered and, if so, to find out how much of the cost you will be responsible for. You may also want to ask about how much will be applied to your deductible, if your deductible has not been met.

- If the amount you expect to be charged is not within your budget, ask your insurance company if there is a way to reduce the cost of the test. Your insurance company may be able to recommend a less expensive testing center within your network. Also ask your doctor whether there is anything they can do. Sometimes a doctor can order the same test but with a different CPT code that will lower the overall cost to you.

- If neither your doctor nor your insurance company can help lower the cost of the test, call around to testing centers to see how much the test would cost out of pocket. Sometimes it is cheaper to pay for tests directly instead of paying through your insurer.

There are also websites that can provide approximate information on costs, such as Clear Health Costs (https://clearhealthcosts.com/) and Healthcare Bluebook (https://www.healthcarebluebook.com/). As much as possible, do your research ahead of time. While the research isn't easy, it's even harder to contest charges once the test has been performed. Doing the legwork ahead of time can save you money and frustration down the road.

Next Steps

By the end of the meeting with your doctor, you should have a concrete sense of your doctor's working diagnosis and what tests they are going to order to confirm or rule out conditions.

Make sure you understand the next steps before you leave. When will the tests be done? When can you expect results? When is the follow-up with the doctor? Understanding the timeline will help reduce stress and also give you a sense of when to call the office if things are not moving along.

The next chapter will explore what to do when your test results come in. Waiting for your test results can be a stressful experience. To the extent that you can, channel any worry or stress into actions that can help you move the process forward. Read up on the tests your doctor ordered so that you feel familiar with what good and bad results look like. Don't assume that no news is good news. Call your doctor's office to follow up on your test results to be sure that no one forgot to call you when they were ready. Let them know that when the results do come in, you'd like to receive a copy so that you can go over them with your doctor. This won't ease your worries entirely, but it will help you stay engaged in the process in a positive way.

Tools for Effective Communication

Your Medical Agenda

What do you want most out of this visit (for example, a diagnosis to explain your symptoms, treatment to relieve pain, help with managing a condition)?

_____

_____

What other things would you like to get out of this visit (for example, a prescription refill, recommendations to improve overall health, advice on other conditions)?

_____

_____

Are there any administrative things that you need out of this visit (for example, signatures on any school- or work-related forms, printed copies of your medical records, booking a future appointment)?

_____

_____

Do you have any assumptions that you have already made about any of the items that you have listed above? For example, if you're hoping that your doctor will give you a diagnosis to explain your symptoms, do you already have an idea based on your online research as to what the diagnosis might be? If you're hoping to improve your overall health, is this because you believe your lifestyle is currently unhealthy? It can be useful to write these notes down on your agenda so you don't forget to raise them with your doctor during your appointment.

_____

_____

_____

Prioritize the agenda items you have listed above. This will help you prioritize the discussion with your doctor and will increase your chance of having all your main points addressed during your appointment.

Scripts

It can sometimes be helpful to have a script to facilitate your conversation with your doctor. We have included phrases below that might be helpful during your appointment.

I'm worried about X symptom because of Y reasons.

The goal here is to be explicit about the symptoms you are most worried about and why. For example, you might say "I'm worried about this headache because I never had one that lasted this long before." Phrasing your thinking this way will give your doctor more context and allow them to directly address your concerns.

I am worried that I have X disease because of Y reasons.

If you are worried about a specific disease, let your doctor know. For example, you might say "I'm worried this lump might be cancerous because my mother had breast cancer when she was young." The added information can help your doctor decide whether the disease you are worried about should be considered as a possible diagnosis.

Could you let me know about your working diagnosis so I understand the situation better?

This helps you understand the doctor's working diagnosis and allows you to do additional research to learn more about the condition.

Is there anything else it could be?

This helps you understand what is on the doctor's list of possibilities (the differential diagnosis).

Is there a reason you are not considering X condition?

This question might help you address any lingering concerns about a diagnosis you are worried about.

Will any of the tests you ordered confirm or rule out the diagnosis?

This gives you more insight into the testing.

Are there any symptoms I should be on the lookout for?

This will give your doctor a chance to let you know about any red flag symptoms, which might require you to seek immediate care.

Should I change anything about my daily routine while we wait for the test results to come in?

This will give your doctor a chance to advise you on immediate changes that might improve your health and, depending on whether your condition is potentially infectious, protect those around you.

Where can I learn more?

Your doctor may be able to provide printed materials or suggest a website.

4 | Receiving a Diagnosis

When your test results come in, you'll likely get a call from your doctor to discuss them. In the best-case scenario, your doctor will give you an all clear and an indication of what to do about your symptoms. But not every situation is that simple.

Ashley Frangipane, a singer better known by her stage name Halsey, recently described her experience being diagnosed with endometriosis.[1] She was twenty years old and sitting in a hotel room in Chicago when she started bleeding uncontrollably. "That night in Chicago, I had a miscarriage," she said, in a speech to supporters at a New York benefit for endometriosis research and education. "I didn't even know I was pregnant and I had a miscarriage and I remember laying in a bed in a hotel room with a towel between my legs, bleeding and staring at my very young, very scared, very male managers who had no idea what was going on."

The miscarriage, though traumatic, led to a discovery that helped answer a question Halsey had been asking herself for years. Ever since she had reached puberty, Halsey had suffered with painful periods that she couldn't explain. "I remember when I had my first job as a hostess at a restaurant," she said. "I remember clearing a table and taking a tray back into the kitchen and collapsing to the floor and rushing to the hospital. There was a lot of misdiagnoses along the way."

One doctor suggested that Halsey may be suffering with a hormonal disorder called polycystic ovary syndrome. Other people in her life told her she was just being sensitive or overdramatic. But no one could give her a full explanation for why she felt the way she did. Until the miscarriage. After her experience in Chicago, Halsey found an obstetrician-gynecologist who helped her determine that the period pain she had been experiencing was a symptom of endometriosis, a chronic condition with no cure but with many treatments that could help her manage the pain.

What some might have expected to be a moment of relief—the moment Halsey received her diagnosis—turned out to be traumatic in its own way. "I didn't know what was going on when I got my diagnosis. I had spent a lifetime tucking my tampons into the sleeve of my sweatshirt when I would go to the bathroom, God forbid anybody knew that I was menstruating because it was like the most shameful thing of all time. And now there was this," she remembered. "I was very fatigued and was fainting backstage at my concerts and I was bleeding and I was pissed off at the whole world. I was like, Why is this happening to me? What did I do to deserve this?"

Those feelings of anger, frustration, and shock are far from uncommon. No matter what your expectations, receiving an unwelcome diagnosis is almost always a shock to the system. In many cases, you may not even be able to process what's being said. This chapter will give you tools that will hopefully help you process your diagnosis and figure out if it fits.

Receiving Your Diagnosis

If you're concerned about what you might hear when you speak with your doctor, consider bringing a friend, family member, or professional health advocate to your appointment (see the box on the next page for information on advocates). If you pick the right person, they can be a supportive force in the room and can help with jotting down information, remembering what was said, and raising points on your agenda that you may overlook in the moment. Many organizations, such as the National Institute on Aging, recommend this approach.[2]

Whether it's someone you know or a hired professional, be careful who you pick. This is an appointment between you and your doctor. You don't want someone in the room who is going to interrupt the flow of the conversation, talk over you or your doctor, or create a defensive or combative environment. There is also likely to be a lot of sensitive personal information shared during the visit, so you'll want to be sure that you're comfortable with your companion hearing the details.

Professional Health Advocates

Professional health advocates help people interact with their health care system, whether that's sitting with them during an appointment, helping them find a doctor for a second opinion, or sorting through medical bills to help them understand what they're being charged for. Advocates come from a variety of backgrounds, and some are former physicians and nurses. Many are simply people whose personal experiences have instilled in them a passion for health advocacy.

Professional health advocacy is a relatively new field, so only a fraction of professional health advocates have become certified through the Patient Advocate Certification Board, which began offering certification in early 2018. The cost of a professional health advocate can vary widely, from as little as $25 per hour to as much as $200 per hour. Advocates sometimes specialize in specific areas, such as dealing with medical bills, or focus on particular conditions, like cancer. Given all this variability, it's important to do your research when choosing a health advocate.

As a starting point, check with your health insurance company or employer to see if there are any relevant benefits that you can take advantage of. If not, you can hire someone directly by searching the Patient Advocate Certification Board website or similar websites, like those of the Patient Advocate Foundation or the National Association of Healthcare Advocacy. The Alliance of Claims Assistance Professionals website can direct you to health advocates who are specialized in medical and insurance claims.

Trisha Torrey, who is featured later in this chapter, started an organization called AdvoConnection to help people link up with professional health advocates. The website (https://advoconnection .com/) has a long list of resources that can help you decide which advocate is right for you. One resource that may prove useful is their list of questions to ask a health advocate before hiring them.[1]

In addition to interviewing potential advocates, it can be helpful to ask for references and speak with people who have previously used the advocate's services. Alternatively, you can see if the advocate offers a free trial or discounted rate so that you can try some of their services without making a full commitment. The available research shows that a good health advocate can improve your interactions with the health care system, but you'll need to do the leg work to find one that fits your needs and your budget.

As emotional as this appointment may become, keep in mind that you have one major goal for this meeting: gathering information. The more you know and understand about your diagnosis, the better off you'll be when you find yourself having to make a decision about what's next.

Use the same tips we described in chapter 3 to prepare for this appointment. Review any notes or questions about your doctor's previous working diagnosis and plan, be prepared to take notes to help you remember the details, and repeat back what you're hearing to be sure you understand what your doctor is saying.

During the appointment itself, the best advice we have is to focus on understanding everything your doctor is trying to tell you: your diagnosis, what your test results mean, and the recommended next steps.

Trusting Your Diagnosis

After the initial emotional shock of an unwelcome diagnosis, there is often a deep yearning for normalcy.[3] In those moments, there really isn't a desire to be an empowered or engaged patient. Most people don't want to be patients at all—they just want the condition or disease to go away so they can go back to being normal.

In some cases, that desire for normalcy translates into an outright rejection of a diagnosis and a belief that the doctor can't possibly be right. The instinct to deny a diagnosis is normal and understandable, but it's not necessarily a healthy one. While there isn't a wealth of evidence in this field, the National Academy of Medicine compiled the available studies and found that the rate of diagnostic error ranges from 5 percent to 17 percent, suggesting that, in the majority of cases, doctors order the right tests, read the results properly, and come to the correct conclusions.[4]

Feeling confident about your doctor's diagnosis and trusting that you have an explanation for the health challenges you've been facing is a liberating experience. Robin Orr is the head of a California-based consulting firm that provides services to health care systems. She knows hospitals inside and out, not just as a professional but also as a patient. Robin had been diagnosed with cancer and overcame it. In 2005, when this particular story took place, she had recently undergone back surgery and had since been suffering with increasing back pain. Late one Friday night, Robin was in such pain that she felt her best option was to go to the ER. She had her care partner with her, a woman named Sue Cook. At the hospital, Robin was given morphine for the pain and a room to rest in for the night.

The next morning, Dr. Eric Trautwein was on duty and came to check on her. Dr. Trautwein is a hospitalist, which is essentially a doctor who cares primarily for hospitalized patients. He didn't know Robin or her medical history, so he did a thorough review of Robin's chart and a detailed examination of her.

"Eric was a breath of fresh air," said Sue in an interview with *The*

Hospitalist magazine later that year.[5] "I'll never forget—he noticed that one knee reflex had a very subtle difference. He wanted to double-check that, saying he never made assumptions. He immediately got tests scheduled for that day, which was a Saturday. That never happens."

Dr. Trautwein scheduled Robin for an immediate CT scan, PET scan, and MRI. By Monday, she had the results: there was a mass behind her abdominal cavity, consistent with metastatic cancer. Without Dr. Trautwein's diligence, the mass could have continued to grow unnoticed for many more months. As Robin put it, "A hospitalist saved my life."

Figuring Out If Your Diagnosis Fits

Robin's story—a trip to the hospital, an examination, tests, and an accurate diagnosis—is thankfully the norm. But there are also rare cases when doctors are wrong about the diagnosis. If you've received your diagnosis and you're concerned that it might be incorrect, there are a few steps you can follow to help you feel more confident about the diagnosis or determine whether you need a second opinion.

Trisha Torrey is a woman who had to figure out these steps on her own. Trisha was watering her garden in upstate New York when she noticed a golf ball–sized lump on her torso. She went online to see if she could figure out what it was. Her search results were all peppered with the word *tumor*, and most sites she visited recommended that she speak with her doctor. She met with her family doctor, who immediately sent her to a surgeon later that day to have the lump removed. After the surgery, the surgeon sent a sample of the lump to a lab for testing.

After an unusually long wait, the surgeon called Trisha to tell her the results. She had a rare cancer called subcutaneous panniculitis-like T-cell lymphoma. It was so unusual, he said, that he had sent the sample to another lab for a second opinion, and both labs independently confirmed the results. When Trisha went online later that day to look up the condition, she could only find two pieces of information that were relevant. "In both cases, I was going to be dead in just a few months," Trisha said.

When Trisha met with her oncologist, he sent her for more blood work and a CT scan, which both came back negative, with no sign of lymphoma and no other abnormalities. She also didn't have any symptoms—her appetite, energy, and overall well-being were as good as they had always been. Still, her doctor insisted that it was possible to feel fine but still have the disease and recommended chemotherapy. "We have results from two labs," her oncologist said. "That's enough to confirm that you've got it."

Even though the oncologist felt confident with the diagnosis, Trisha knew something wasn't right. She fought to get a copy of her test results and decided to dig deeper into what they meant. When she came up against a word or a test that she didn't understand, she looked it up online. By the end of her search, she felt that she had a rough understanding of what her results meant, and she was more convinced than ever that she was on the right track and her doctors had misread the results.

"In the meantime, my oncologist was calling me every day to try to get a port for the chemotherapy medications installed," Trisha said. "'You're not dying on my watch!' is what he would say to me. It was a very, very difficult time."

By chance, Trisha had a friend who knew an oncologist named Dr. Jeffrey Kirchner. After meeting with Trisha and hearing her story, he suggested that they send a specimen from her lump to a pathologist at the National Institutes of Health who had dealt with this rare type of lymphoma before. In September, three months after Trisha had found the lump, she received the results saying that there was no malignancy. She never had cancer.

Without even knowing it, Trisha had done what researchers say is the most effective way to figure out if a diagnosis fits and reduce the chance of misdiagnosis—she became informed and worked with her doctor as part of the diagnostic team. Since her misdiagnosis, she has gone on to work in patient advocacy to help others learn how to do the same thing (see the box earlier in the chapter). "Now I say to the patients I talk to, 'Your hour on the internet does not equal twelve years of medical education and experience. But if you approach your doctor by asking questions respectfully, based on the information you've found, most doctors will discuss it with you. And if they don't, find yourself another doctor.'"

Think Like Your Doctor: Becoming Part of the Diagnostic Team

The National Academy of Medicine published a report on reducing misdiagnosis.[4] One of its primary recommendations is for patients to become part of the diagnostic team. As the authors of the report put it, "The diagnostic process hinges on successful collaboration among health care professionals, patients, and their families. Patients and their families are critical partners in the diagnostic process."

Research Your Diagnosis

Taking an active role in your diagnosis starts with understanding it. Go online and ask yourself whether the diagnosis you've been given sounds right to you. Do the symptoms you listed on your symptom tracker fit the condition? Does the condition have other symptoms that don't line up with yours? Do you fit the profile of a typical person with the condition?

One thing you'll need to understand is where you fall on the spectrum of the disease. If you are in the early stages of the condition, your symptoms may be very different than what you would expect if you were at a more advanced stage. You want to be sure that your symptoms line up with the diagnosis but also that the progression of your symptoms matches what is expected.

To the extent that you can, try to keep your emotions out of the picture. A doctor's communication style and bedside manner can have a significant impact on how much you trust a diagnosis. There is a body of research on the role of emotions in the health care context. For example, people are much less likely to sue a doctor that they have a good relationship with, as opposed to one they don't like.[6] Similarly, inadequate doctor-patient communication is a significant factor in patients seeking second opinions.[7,8] The bottom line is that it's important to be aware of the emotional component as you think through whether your diagnosis fits. Using objective approaches like comparing your symptom tracker with the information online can help avoid this pitfall.

Figuring out whether a diagnosis fits is a hard thing to do, especially for people with no medical training. If, after objective research, something doesn't seem right to you, start digging deeper into your test results.

Obtain Copies of Your Test Results

If you didn't automatically receive a copy of your test results before or during your appointment, ask your doctor for a copy. Some providers may hesitate to share too much detail with you, but getting a copy of your medical records is well within your rights. In 1996, the Health Insurance Portability and Accountability Act (HIPAA) clarified people's right to receive and review their health information, which includes their medical records and bills.[9] This can be one of the most important things you can do to take control of your health. Not only will it help you understand your diagnosis in the short term, it will also help you over the long term if you find that you need to coordinate care between multiple doctors in the future.

While health care facilities can charge you a nominal fee for the labor required to make a copy of your records, they are not allowed to deny you access even if you have unpaid bills. Be aware though that medical records can sometimes be hundreds of pages long, particularly if you have had multiple hospitalizations. It may be prudent to specify the most relevant records for your needs, or ask whether your records are available electronically. Increasingly, medical centers are making records available free of charge through online patient portals. However, if you have a complicated condition, your imaging tests (such as CT scans and MRIs) may not be available through the portal, and you may want to ask for copies of the images to be shared with you separately.

Learn What Your Test Results Mean

Once you have your test results, dive into what the results mean, even if the process feels daunting. A basic starting point is to go through the results and figure out what the acronyms refer to and what the more complex terminology means. You're not trying to get to the same level of understanding of these results as your doctor, you're just trying to get comfortable with the overall gist of the results.[10]

> Note the tests that show a **negative or normal** result. This means that the condition or substance tested for was not found. It might seem counterintuitive, but a negative result is usually a good thing as it means no abnormalities were found.
>
> If a test shows a **positive or abnormal** result, it means that the condition or substance was found, and you're going to want to follow up on these tests in more detail.
>
> Anything that is **inconclusive or uncertain** means that there wasn't enough information to diagnose or rule out the condition. You're likely going to want to talk to your doctor in more detail about results like these.

One thing to keep in mind is the possibility of false positives and false negatives. A false positive means that your test shows you have a disease or condition, but you don't actually have it. A false negative means that the results say you're all clear, but in fact you do actually have the disease or condition. Incorrect results don't happen often, but they are more likely with certain types of tests or if the testing was not done correctly. You can search online to determine whether the test you had has a higher or lower chance of delivering incorrect results. Search for things like "accuracy of X test" or "chances of false positive/negative for X test." Keep in mind that the accuracy of some tests depends on whether you are male or female, so consider adding that in the search string.

While you're well within your rights to ask to undergo a test again, be aware that many doctors—knowing how accurate tests generally are—will assume that your request for another test is coming from an emotional place and an inability to accept the diagnosis. Make sure you do your research well before making the request. Understanding your symptoms, diagnosis, and why your test results don't fit will help you have an informed discussion with your doctor and help explain your desire to be tested again. We have included scripts at the end of this chapter that may be helpful when you talk through your concerns with your doctor.

Decide Whether to Pursue a Second Opinion

If, after all your research and after speaking with your doctor about your concerns, you and your doctor still aren't on the same page about your diagnosis, consider a second opinion. Given the intimate nature of the patient-doctor relationship, it can feel uncomfortable to ask another doctor for a second opinion. However, it is a perfectly acceptable practice. It may not even involve a visit to another doctor. In recent years, many leading hospitals have started remote second opinion services, offering to send your relevant medical records to a remote expert who can provide an opinion on the diagnosis and treatment.

When looking for another doctor to assess your condition, consider where the doctor was trained, their board certifications, online ratings or reviews, and any malpractice history. In the United States, malpractice history is posted publicly on state medical board websites. You can find a list of state medical boards and their websites via the Federation of State Medical Boards (https://www.fsmb.org/). When you read through online reviews, keep in mind that many people choose doctors based on how they interact with them rather than on ratings or reviews.[11] Read reviews carefully to see why a doctor is being recommended and whether their positive attributes line up with what you need. You also want to look for their number of years of practice, particularly when you need a procedure. Research suggests that longer experience is associated with better outcomes.[12] And don't forget to check with your insurance company before booking the appointment so that you understand what the expected costs of a second opinion with the doctor you select might be.

If you are concerned about a specific condition or, like Trisha, you've been diagnosed with something that is uncommon, try to find a doctor who specializes in that condition. Look for doctors affiliated with an academic center since they tend to be experts in their field. Their level of expertise should hopefully give you more confidence in their opinion.

When you go to an appointment for a second opinion, make sure to take your medical records with you. It might be tempting to not tell the doctor anything about your previous diagnosis in an effort to not bias their opinion, but holding back information may put you at risk of the doorknob phenomenon we talked about earlier, where concerns about your previous diagnosis may not be addressed until the very end of the appointment or at all. Instead, we encourage you to be open and direct when seeking a second opinion. Let the doctor know what you were diagnosed with, why you're concerned the diagnosis doesn't fit, and that you're looking for a second opinion. After letting the doctor know your expectations upfront, you can let them do their job. Allow the doctor time to do their assessment and then ask any questions you still have. As one research study eloquently noted, "Second opinion encounters may be beneficial if physicians and patients communicate openly, positively and respectfully."[13]

When There Is No Diagnosis

In some cases, there will be no diagnosis. This can be an incredibly frustrating conclusion to a stressful situation. There is no easy answer or guidance for what to do in this situation, except to keep at it. Go back to your original list of possible conditions that you created from your initial online search, and do more research on some of the more obscure conditions. Consider joining online forums for those conditions and asking others if they went undiagnosed for a while.

There are a number of support groups and organizations that may also be able to help. For example, Syndromes Without A Name, or SWAN, is a nonprofit organization dedicated to supporting children and young adults who have symptoms without a diagnosis. The National Institutes of Health Common Fund has set up the Undiagnosed Diseases Network, a study that brings together research and medical centers across the United States that are working to improve the diagnosis and care of people with undiagnosed diseases. Organizations like these can be an important source of support.

Some small research studies suggest that crowdsourcing tools might help,[14,15] but others are more cautionary.[16] With online programs such as CrowdMed, people submit their cases and case solvers sign up to help diagnose them. *The New York Times* has a "Diagnosis" column where Dr. Lisa Sanders features people with an unsolved medical mystery and asks readers to help determine the diagnosis. Crowdsourcing options are still new and relatively untested, so be wary about accepting any results from this approach without doing additional research.

Whenever you find new information that you think might be valuable in helping you determine your condition, share it with your doctor. The doctor will help you make sense of the information and put it into context, and together you may ultimately get to a diagnosis.

Talking to Your Doctor about Your Concerns

You might consider starting the conversation with your doctor by trying to get a better understanding of why your doctor made the diagnosis:

> *Could you walk me through how you came to this diagnosis?*
> *Do the test results fit the diagnosis?*
> *Do all of my symptoms fit the diagnosis?*
> *Are there any symptoms that don't fit?*

Once you have a better sense of why your doctor made the diagnosis, try to find out what other conditions they considered or may still be considering:

> *Is there anything else you think/thought it could be?*
> *Could there be more than one thing going on?*

If you disagree with your doctor about a condition—your doctor has ruled it out but you believe that they may be wrong—or there's a condition that your doctor didn't mention but that you fear you have, approach the situation respectfully while explaining your concerns:

> *I'm really trying to stay engaged in this process, so I've been*
> *doing some research.*
> *I'm worried I could have X condition for Y reasons.*
> *What do you think?*

If you get pushback from your doctor about going online to do research, try not to respond defensively and instead engage your doctor in the process by asking them if there are websites or other sources of information where you can turn to find out more about the conditions that are worrying you. Be polite but persistent to get the answers to your questions and have your concerns addressed.

5 | Deciding on Treatment

When Kapil and I reached this chapter in the book, I asked him if he wouldn't mind if I started this one on my own. If you read the prologue, you know a bit about the story of my husband and I trying to navigate cancer treatment options far from friends and family and in a country where we didn't speak the language.

One appointment always stands out for me. My husband's doctors wanted his treatment to start immediately but had warned us that it could lead to infertility. At the time, we had one amazing little girl, but we were hoping to have another child if we could. We asked the doctors if we could speak to a specialist to find out more, so they quickly secured an appointment for us with two fertility doctors. We explained, through an interpreter, that we wanted to pursue the treatment but that we also wanted to have more kids. The doctors told us unequivocally that if we started the cancer treatment, we would never be able to have more children. "One hundred percent, no children possible," they told us.

We were stunned so asked again to be sure, "One hundred percent?" "Yes," they said. "But use protection to be sure." None of it made any sense to us. We went home and spent the next few days reading as much as we could online about my husband's treatments. We also tried searching other fertility options, to see if there was another approach that could work for us. All the while, we were being pressured by our doctors, who only wanted the best for my husband, to decide quickly when he would start treatment.

We felt like we were being rushed through some very major, life-altering decisions. We were emotional, scared, and desperate for life to return to normal, and this led us to make some decisions too quickly, without being fully informed. This chapter is for anyone out there who has felt the same or who has a loved one going through the same process. Hopefully, the chapter will teach you some important ways to slow down decision-making in these crucial moments so that you can make the best choice for you and the people around you.

Identifying Your Goals

Health systems are designed, for the most part, to cure, prevent, or manage disease. As a result, doctors often set goals for their patients that are strictly focused on health. Our goals as individuals, however, are much broader than our health. There is a body of scientific litera-ture that suggests that even subtle differences in goals may be mean-ingful for the care you receive,[1] so it's important that you and your doctor are on the same page about your personal goals before deciding on a treatment.

Consider a very minor condition. Let's say you sprain your ankle the day before your daughter's graduation. It's a minor ankle sprain, so your doctor recommends the standard treatment: rest, ice, compres-sion, and elevation for two to three days. A person concerned only about physical health would skip the graduation and rest at home. But most of us don't work that way. Our desire to be there for our child would likely outweigh the risk of not resting the ankle all day. Talking with your doctor about your personal goals and how they relate to your health gives you the opportunity to find the treatment options that best fit you and your life.

To help you think through what's important to you and how it relates to your health, research suggests the following categories to consider.[2]

Functional status: This describes your activity level and how your body functions. What level of functionality would you aspire to or, in the worst-case scenario, could you tolerate? If you have always wanted to run a marathon, for example, then your functional status goal might be more advanced than someone who has no such desire.

Symptoms: This refers to the control of symptoms. Think of common symptoms like nausea, pain, fatigue, or shortness of breath. How willing are you to live with uncomfortable symptoms? Sometimes total elimination is the goal, but other times some degree of pain or other symptom is acceptable.

Life prolongation: This refers to the length of our lives. What are your thoughts and feelings around how long you want to live? Some of us have a specific goal in mind when it comes to how long we want to live. We might want to live for as long as possible, assuming we are independent and healthy, or we might have a milestone moment in mind like seeing our grandkids graduate from college.

Well-being: This refers to a more general sense of wellness. What do you need in your life to make you feel relaxed and happy? Goals related to well-being, such as having purpose and meaning in life or avoiding stress and anxiety, are often very closely related to our health.

Work or social responsibilities: This dimension deals more specifically with our interactions with other people. A person may have a family to support or may be caring for a child or parent in need. What is the level of support that is best for you and those around you?

Thinking through these categories as you define your personal health goals will help you and your doctor weigh the pros and cons of various treatment options.

Deciding Whether Treatment Is Necessary

One helpful thing about using a goal-centered approach is that it can offer an opportunity to think about whether treatment is needed at all. Sometimes, the benefits of treatment are not sufficiently important for your goals, or the treatment is too burdensome. There's no single rule or checklist to follow to make this decision, but there are some situations when you might want to think seriously about the possibility of not accepting treatment.

End-Stage Diseases

As its name suggests, having an end-stage disease is essentially being in the final phase of a progressive condition. If you or someone you love has been diagnosed with an end-stage disease, you will be grappling with a lot of conflicting emotions and many tough choices. For some people, treatment for an end-stage disease may only gain them a few additional months of life and maybe not even a high quality of life depending on how invasive and uncomfortable the treatment may be.

The value of treatment is often made clear by asking a question about the natural history of the condition, like "What is the course of the disease with no treatment?" In some cases, such as a heart attack, treatment can be lifesaving. With hypertension, not choosing treatment can lead to major damage to multiple organs, including the eyes and kidneys. But in other cases, like Alzheimer's disease, the impact of treatment on the overall course of the disease is much more modest. You can find general information about the course of a disease online, but your doctor will be able to tell you more about your specific situation.

We talk more about making decisions related to end-of-life matters in chapter 10 and provide additional context and information that can help you think through your choices if you are diagnosed with an end-stage disease. You may find, after careful consideration of your treatment options and goals, that choosing no treatment is the best path to follow.

Early-Stage and Mild Diseases

On the other side of the spectrum are early-stage and mild diseases. In the same way that you might not rush to the doctor's office if you get the sniffles, you may not want to rush into treatment if your condition is still in the earliest stages.

Let's say you've been diagnosed with mitral regurgitation. This is a condition in which the mitral valve in your heart doesn't fully close, so blood leaks back into the heart instead of being pumped out. It's a serious condition that can sometimes lead to heart failure and even death. If your condition is severe, heart surgery is by far your best option. But heart surgery comes with a range of side effects, including emotional, financial, and medical. If you're diagnosed with mild mitral regurgitation, you may not want to jump to treatment so quickly. In situations like this, it might just be better to wait and see how things develop. This approach has a medical name—*watchful waiting*.[3]

With watchful waiting, you and your doctor agree to monitor your condition closely together. If things worsen, you reassess the possibility of treatment. If things stay the same, you continue monitoring for any possible changes. In some cases, the condition may resolve on its own.

While it can be tempting to think, "What's the harm in treating the condition?" or "Why wait and take a chance?" remember that medical procedures and treatments can have serious side effects. In some situations, these negative effects may exceed any benefit that comes from treating the condition. There may also be public health consequences to undergoing unnecessary treatments. For example, overprescription of antibiotics has resulted in resistant strains of bacteria,[4] which can be a problem not just for you but for others in the community.

Watchful waiting might make sense for some conditions like certain early-stage cancers that are known to be very slow growing. It could also be useful in situations like ear infections in children or back pain in adults. Keep in mind though that watchful waiting is not the same as doing nothing. Being vigilant and monitoring your symptoms for possible progression of the disease is an important part of watchful waiting.

Think Like Your Doctor: Review Your Recommended Treatment against the Guidelines

If you think you're likely to pursue treatment, investigate your treatment options. Regardless of whether they are lifestyle changes, medications, or procedures, almost all treatments offered are based on an approach called evidence-based medicine.[5] What this means is that the treatments are chosen based on their efficacy, or effectiveness, in research studies.

For many conditions and diseases, groups of experts meet to review all the relevant scientific studies and work together to develop treatment guidelines. The guidelines are available to individual physicians who can then use them to inform how they treat their patients, adapting them as needed for each individual case. The guidelines aren't perfect,[6] but they're still quite helpful for doctors. It's as though all the Major League Baseball coaches wrote up what they all agreed were the best coaching strategies. Imagine having that document when coaching a little league team—it could really help improve performance.

While the guidelines are targeted to doctors, it is often helpful for people to review the treatment their doctor recommended against the guidelines to see if they align. Treatment guidelines are complex, technical documents written for health care professionals, but sometimes there are patient-friendly summaries. Even if there isn't one available, it might still be worth taking the time to review the treatment recommendations for the condition you've been diagnosed with. At the end of this chapter, we've included a list of sources for treatment guidelines to help you in your search.

The most important recommendations to focus on are the strongest ones. For example, the GRADE (Grading of Recommendations, Assessment, Development and Evaluation) system was developed as a way to describe the strength of recommendations.[7] The ratings range from "high," which is associated with a lot of confidence, to "very low." In this case, it would be prudent to focus on the recommendations with a "high" GRADE rating.

Other guidelines use a class of recommendation as well as quality of evidence. For example, heart disease guidelines typically have a "class or strength of recommendation" as well as a "level of evidence" associated with each recommendation. Class I recommendations are for treatments that offer a substantial benefit. Class IIb recommendations are considered weak recommendations, meaning the treatment offers only a slight benefit. The level of evidence grade refers to how much research exists on the treatment. Level A means there is high-quality evidence from multiple randomized controlled trials, whereas Level C indicates a low level of evidence.

If you were diagnosed with heart disease, you would want to make sure your doctor had recommended a Class I treatment with Level A evidence. If so, you can feel confident that you're following a treatment plan that has strong scientific support. If your treatment doesn't line up, don't worry unnecessarily. Instead, use it as an opportunity to be a more engaged partner in your own treatment plan, and ask your doctor to explain their reasoning.

Research suggests that as many as 40 percent of people in the United States and around the world don't get the treatments that are recommended by professional guidelines.[8] This happens for a variety of reasons.[9] In a few cases, the person has some risk factor that makes the recommended treatment inappropriate. In other cases, it is due to accidental oversight or insufficient awareness on the part of the doctor. By raising the issue of treatment guidelines with your doctor, you'll help prevent any oversight.

If you do raise the issue, be respectful, but upfront and honest. If possible, mention the professional body as the source and inquire if the guidelines apply to you. For example, "I was reading that the American College of Cardiology recommends a blood thinner for atrial fibrillation. Do you think that's right for me?" The answer from your doctor should give you a sense of their clinical reasoning.

The next four chapters will explore the main categories of treatment: medications, surgical procedures, lifestyle changes, and complementary and alternative treatments. Each treatment category requires a unique approach to determine whether any of the treatment options available to you are the right fit.

Treatment Guidelines

Many treatment guidelines are available online. The US Centers for Disease Control and Prevention has an online database of guidelines and recommendations for hundreds of diseases and conditions (https://stacks.cdc.gov/cbrowse?pid=cdc%3A100&parentId=cdc%3A100). The website of the National Institute for Clinical Excellence in the United Kingdom houses a similar database (https://www.guidelines.co.uk/).

The American Academy of Family Physicians database includes guidelines for many conditions affecting children, adolescents, and adults (https://www.aafp.org/patient-care/browse/type.tag-clinical-practice-guidelines.html). For guidelines related to children's diseases, visit the American Academy of Pediatrics website (https://www.healthychildren.org/English/Pages/default.aspx).

For guidelines related specifically to heart disease, check the website of the American Heart Association (https://www.heart.org/)

or the American College of Cardiology (https://www.cardiosmart .org/). For cancer guidelines, visit the National Comprehensive Cancer Network (https://www.nccn.org/).

If you can't find clinical practice guidelines for the condition you're looking for but want to know what treatment approaches experts recommend, consider signing up for a professional medical resource such as UpToDate (https://www.uptodate.com/home) or DynaMed (https://www.dynamed.com/). These tools, like the guidelines, are intended for doctors, so it will require a fair bit of work for the average person to fully understand the content.

Another valuable resource is the library at a large hospital where the staff have access to a wide range of patient and professional health resources. You may be able to get help finding treatment recommendations online.

As you do your research, it's important to keep in mind that all these guidelines and resources are not a substitute for medical advice, but rather one more way to become more informed about your condition so that you can discuss your treatment options with your doctor.

6 | Medications

By far the most common treatment prescribed by doctors is some kind of medication, taken by mouth, inhaled, or applied as a cream. Despite how common prescriptions are, people don't always fill them or take them as recommended. Sometimes, it's a matter of logistics. Costs may be prohibitive, or refills are not provided on time, so we stop taking a medicine that we know could improve our health. Other times, it's more emotional. We may resist the idea of taking a medication for the rest of our lives, or we feel that we can't accept the side effects or other implications of taking the drug.

It is possible, though, to work together with your doctor to make the most of what medications have to offer while minimizing the negative effects. Take Whitney Petit for example.[1] Diagnosed with epilepsy in childhood, her disease became dormant, and she was seizure free for seventeen years. Then, when she was twenty-seven years old, she had another seizure. Her doctor immediately started her on 1,000 mg of a popular seizure medication called levetiracetam (brand name Keppra). It took about a week before Whitney began noticing unwelcome changes in her body. She couldn't wake up in the mornings and would sleep in until noon, she couldn't control her emotions and would find herself in fits of rage, and the biggest one, at least for her at the time, was that she started to lose her hair. All this, and she was still having seizures.

When she went in for her follow-up, her doctor listened to her concerns but still recommended increasing her dosage to 2,000 mg and eventually suggested adding a second drug. For many of us, that might have been the breaking point—the moment when we decided to either stop taking the medications or succumb to the inevitable and simply accept the consequences. But Whitney took a different route. She decided that she would see what else she could do to limit the side effects and potentially free herself from medications altogether.

Whitney chronicled her journey online. "After each seizure I kept a log of what was happening prior to the seizure," she wrote. "These logs helped me to identify my seizure triggers. My triggers include lack of sleep, too much sleep, changes in the weather such as quick pressure drops, certain foods like fresh apples and aspartame, stress, my hormones and of course heat." Once she knew her triggers, she worked with her doctor and other specialists to try to reduce their impact. She started on a ketogenic diet,[2] transitioned to natural food products to reduce the aluminum in her body, and added vitamins to her daily cocktail of medications.[3] Eventually, she was able to limit her seizures to about one a month, and her doctor took her off Keppra completely.

One of the key lessons in Whitney's story is that it doesn't have to be an all or nothing approach when it comes to medications. It's not a matter of just taking a medication and tolerating unbearable side effects. Nor is it abandoning medications altogether. It's about working with your doctor to make the best of the situation based on the available information.

Shared Decision-Making

With this chapter of the book, we hope to give you a set of tools to help you work with your doctor to decide whether the right treatment plan for you includes medications. The process, called shared decision-making, can be used to make choices about many different types of treatment, but here we focus specifically on medications. Shared decision-making involves doctors and patients working together to make decisions about which medications can improve a patient's health outcomes while balancing those outcomes against the patient's preferences and overall well-being.

While the approach has become increasingly popular in recent years,[4] it's not always put into practice, often because doctors and patients don't have the time to explore these decisions in detail together. In most cases, doctors understand a vast amount of information about the drugs that they prescribe, but the average appointment is far too short to share all this information with a patient.

Generally, your doctor is focused on explaining the benefits of the drug, helping you understand why it could be an important part of your treatment plan, and talking through the most common side effects or the ones most relevant to you. Delving into the pros and cons of one type of medication versus another or exploring the full list of side effects associated with any single medication isn't likely to happen during your visit. This isn't due to a lack of care or compassion on the doctor's part, but rather to the constraints of time—a reality that both doctors and patients must face in today's health care system. With this in mind, patients have to be proactive and prepared in order to get to shared decision-making.

Ask the Right Questions

To begin with, if your doctor prescribes a medication, make sure that you fully understand its benefits. This is something that your doctor is in a unique position to explain, given their medical understanding of your condition, the medication, and their rationale for prescribing it. Some questions can help you get a better understanding of this rationale:

- How will this medication affect my condition? Is it meant to cure the condition completely or just keep it under control?
- How effective is the drug?

- Is the drug likely to be more effective or less effective than usual given my particular situation?
- When should I expect my symptoms to go away?
- What do I do if my symptoms don't go away when they are expected to?

Then, it's time to consider the other side of the equation—the risks. The most common concern people have about taking a medication is related to the side effects, that is, the unintended effects that a drug may have. If there is any chance that you might be pregnant, be sure to mention this to your doctor because some medications can cause severe birth defects. The following questions can help you work through this part of the discussion with your doctor:

- What are the most common side effects of the medication?
- What are the most serious side effects? Am I particularly at risk for any of these?
- Will I need any monitoring, like blood tests?
- What should I do if I think I am experiencing any of these side effects?
- Will it interact with any of the other medications I am taking?

Once you feel comfortable with the benefits and risks of the medication your doctor has prescribed, it's time to ask key questions that will help you decide whether or not you should take the medication at all:

- What would happen if I didn't take this medication?
- What would happen if I waited before starting the medication?

- Are there any other treatments that might be an option if I decide not to take this medication?

As we have mentioned in other chapters, take notes during the discussion since they will help you when you do your research later.

Explore Your Doctor's Advice at Home

Once you've gathered the important information from your doctor, it's worthwhile to do some follow-up research on the medications you were prescribed. As you start looking up information online, be aware of the risk of misinformation. Some foundational concepts might be helpful here as you go about your search.

Researching Benefits

Many websites will mention the diseases that medications treat but do not talk specifically about the effectiveness of the medications. This is partly because it can be hard to quantify the exact impact of the medication on the disease, particularly for medications used to treat rare conditions. Even when the evidence is available, explaining it to people can be challenging. If there are many studies on the topic, there may be different findings that have to be reconciled, and the statistics that describe how well a drug works aren't easily understood. One strategy that could help is to look at clinical guidelines and expert opinions as we described in chapter 5. Another option is to see if there are any decision aids for the specific medication you are exploring. These are tools that can help summarize the complex information on the effectiveness of drugs.[5]

Researching Side Effects

Generally speaking, the lists of side effects for drugs are long and exhaustive. Take aspirin, for example, a relatively common over-the-counter drug. Reputable websites will almost always list all the potential side effects, even extremely rare ones that also happen to be among the most frightening, such as internal bleeding or going into shock from an allergic reaction. While it's important for doctors to know all the possible reactions to the drug, the long list of side effects can sometimes dissuade someone from taking the drug. When looking at the list of side effects, it might be more helpful to focus on the common ones. If there are any side effects that you are particularly concerned about, you can look into how often they are reported. In the case of aspirin, the risk of an allergic reaction ranges from 0.01 percent to 0.1 percent. In contrast, indigestion is more common, at about 1 percent to 10 percent.

Researching Pain Control

The opioid crisis in the United States put a spotlight on pain medications and the balance between controlling pain and overprescribing medications that can lead to addiction and overdosing. As a result, there are many people who now question the value of taking any pain medication at all. There are other options to control pain, from non-narcotic painkillers to nondrug approaches such as mindfulness, deep breathing, and even electrical stimulation. In some cases, opioid medications are necessary and can be used responsibly. While a deep dive into pain medication options is beyond the scope of this book, we encourage you to be aware of the risks and research your pain control options. If you have any concerns about taking opioid medications, discuss them in detail with your doctor.

Researching Interactions

Many medications interact with other medications, and it is important to be mindful of this. Usually, electronic medical records and pharmacy computer systems detect interactions between medications automatically, but there are online tools if you want to double-check. Oftentimes, people don't realize that over-the-counter medications can have interactions with their prescribed medications. Your pharmacist is a great resource for helping you determine if any of your medications may interact. Many medications also interact with alcohol or foods, such as grapefruit juice. A quick check online or a discussion with a pharmacist can help prevent any issues.

Resolve Unanswered Questions

If, after your online search, you still have concerns about your medication, schedule a visit with your doctor to explain your thinking and decide together on other possible treatment options. Have an agenda ready, and print off any supporting material that you feel may be useful for the discussion. If possible, frame the discussion in a collaborative manner rather than putting your doctor in a defensive position. You might try saying something like, "I am concerned about X medication for Y reasons. Here is what my research shows, but I'd love to know what you think and work together to find a solution."

The more specific you can be during this discussion, the better. Being specific will allow your doctor to address your concerns and explain how the medication applies to your individual situation. A general statement such as, "I'm worried about the side effects" is likely to lead to a general response like, "The side effects are generally mild" or "Serious side effects are rare," both of which are true statements but probably information you already knew.

Another resource that is often underutilized is a pharmacist. You can schedule a visit with your pharmacist or just walk into the pharmacy and ask for a few minutes of their time. Some pharmacies also give you options for interacting with the pharmacist by email or phone instead. Generally speaking, it's a good idea to keep your doctor in the loop with any medication changes recommended by the pharmacist.

Taking Your Medications

If you've decided to fill your prescription and take a new medication, there are some practical steps to follow. First, determine how you're meant to take your medication—what time of day, with food or without, and for how many days.

Once you know the basics, create a routine to help you remember to take your drugs properly. Research shows that many people occasionally skip doses or don't finish all the medication.[6] This is a challenge since you may not get the full benefits of the drug or it may not work at all. There is a wealth of information on how to be more consistent with taking medications.[7] One of the most effective methods is to tie taking the drug with an existing routine. For example, if you brush your teeth just before going to bed and you can take the drug without food, then place your medication with your toothbrush. If you need to take your medication with food, consider putting the pills in the kitchen or packing them with your lunch.

A weekly or monthly pillbox can make it easier when you need to take multiple medications. It can also help when you can't recall if you took all the medication for the day. If you do end up skipping a dose, call your doctor's office or talk to your pharmacist to figure out what you should do. For many medications, they'll tell you to take the next scheduled dose, but if you end up missing multiple doses, you need to be more careful.

Much like when you first started to feel ill, it's important to track your symptoms so you know if the medication is improving your condition and whether you are experiencing any new symptoms that could be due to side effects. It will also help you avoid what's called the *nocebo effect*. Like the more commonly known *placebo effect*—where a person believes that they are taking a treatment and that belief alone is enough for their condition to improve—the nocebo effect is what happens when a person believes they'll experience negative effects from a drug and then start to experience those symptoms because of this thinking. Keeping track of both symptom improvement and side effects may help offset the nocebo effect.

If you do develop side effects, it is vital that you talk to your doctor. In one study, only about half of the people who identified potential side effects reported them to their doctor.[8] By speaking with your doctor, you can decide together ways to reduce the side effects that you're experiencing. Sometimes changing the dose or timing of the medication can help. In other cases, the doctor may be able to suggest lifestyle changes or other drugs to help. If the side effect is particularly bothersome or concerning, have a discussion about whether it's worth continuing to take the drug.

Paying for Medications

For many people, the cost of medications can be quite high, even with health insurance. Because of the way the system is set up, we often don't know how expensive the drug will be until we're at the cash register.

If the cost of your drug is too high, consider asking the pharmacist to ring it up without insurance because it might be cheaper. One study analyzed the prices that 1.6 million people paid for 9.5 million prescriptions and found that 23 percent actually paid more with insurance than if they had paid for it entirely out of pocket.[9] You can also ask if there is a generic version of the drug that costs less. If these options don't work, you can try shopping around. Websites such as GoodRx (https://www.goodrx.com/) and Blink Health (https://www.blinkhealth.com/) allow you to compare costs across different pharmacies for drugs that you are paying for out of pocket. If you are using insurance, you might need to bring your prescription into each different pharmacy so the staff can estimate the costs.

In some cases, you may be able to take advantage of legitimate online options that offer convenient home delivery. However, you should be aware that there are numerous scams and rogue pharmacies online.

The Food and Drug Administration cautions that these pharmacies often sell medicines that don't contain the correct ingredients.[10] They offer guidance for people searching for online pharmacies and suggest avoiding pharmacies that allow you to buy prescription medicines without a valid prescription, pharmacies that are located outside the United States and don't have a US state–licensed pharmacist available to answer your questions, and pharmacies that offer very low prices that seem too good to be true.

Another option to explore is online patient assistance programs developed by pharmaceutical companies. These can provide substantial savings, particularly with medications that are very expensive. Finally, if you have a Flexible Spending Account or Health Savings Account, you may be able to apply money from these accounts toward your prescription medication costs.

The bottom line is that being proactive could result in significant savings that add up over time.

7 | Surgery

Leah Leilani is no stranger to hospitals. Diagnosed with a rare muscle disorder in childhood, she had been in and out of hospitals more times than she could count. When Leah was a teenager, she was told she needed a relatively simple surgery to treat sores in her throat. The surgery was such a simple one that Leah and her family chose to have it done at a surgicenter, which is essentially an outpatient facility with no emergency medical center on site. It should have been a routine procedure, but partway through, Leah's body temperature started to rise and her heart rate escalated. Her parents, who were sitting in the waiting room, were rushed into a separate room and handed a Do Not Resuscitate form—they were being asked whether Leah should be resuscitated if her heart stopped while she was on the surgical table.

At the time, Leah's parents feared that she wouldn't come out of the surgicenter alive. In the operating room, the doctors were realizing that Leah's reaction may be the result of a condition called malignant hyperthermia. When people with malignant hyperthermia are exposed to certain anesthetics, they can have severe muscle spasms and their body temperature and heart rate can rise to dangerously high levels. It's a life-threatening condition, and one that Leah didn't even know she had.

Thankfully, as a result of the quick work of the doctors in the room, Leah survived her surgery, though the emotional trauma to Leah and her parents lingered.[1] While Leah's story is indeed rare, fears and concerns about having surgery, or "going under the knife," are all too common. This chapter explores the steps you can take if your doctor has recommended surgery as a treatment and offers tools to help you prepare for the surgery and have a successful recovery.

Unfortunately, there are some critical emergency situations that require an immediate surgical response. In those cases, there is little that you or the people around you can do to prepare in advance. The only guidance we offer for those situations is to follow the advice of the emergency doctors. Their training and experience are what will save your life, and the best thing you can do is make it as easy as possible for them to do their work, without any interference that could cause unnecessary delays.

Deciding on Surgery

Many of the tools we've shared in other chapters of this book apply to your decision about whether or not to agree to surgery. First, make sure that you understand the benefits and effectiveness of the surgery versus other treatment options. It could help to ask questions like "What happens if I don't get the surgery?" or "Are there any other treatment options?" to really understand how the surgery will affect your condition.

You also want to have a strong understanding of the risks associated with the surgery, including potential organ damage, scarring, and even the level of pain you will experience after the surgery. Consider asking specifically about whether you are at an increased risk for complications due to your age or other medical conditions. Weighing these risks against the benefits, and in the context of the treatment goals we described in chapter 5, is an important step before agreeing to any surgical procedure.

One approach that has been rigorously tested is to ask your doctor about the best-case and worst-case scenarios of the surgery and where you likely fall between these two extremes. Then, ask the same question if you were to not have the surgery—what would be the best outcome if you didn't have the surgery, and what would be the worst that could happen. At the end of this chapter, we've adapted a version of this decision aid that you can use to facilitate this discussion with your doctor.

Decision aids have been created for hundreds of surgical and nonsurgical procedures, for conditions ranging from cancer and heart disease to arthritis and asthma. Many of them can be found with a simple online search with the name of your condition and "decision aid." The Ottawa Hospital Research Institute currently houses a long list of decision aids on their website.[2]

Generally speaking, we encourage you to trust your doctor's guidance, but never blindly. One thing to keep in mind, for example, is the type of doctor who recommended the surgery. As you might imagine, surgeons are more likely to recommend surgery than nonsurgeons. In the case of back pain, a primary care doctor or rheumatologist may have a series of nonsurgical options that they would want to try before surgery, whereas an orthopedic surgeon may recommend a surgical procedure much sooner. Similarly, a cardiologist may be less likely to recommend surgery to treat a heart condition compared to a cardiothoracic surgeon.

There can also be great variability between surgeons. In one study, surgeons were asked to review cases and decide if surgery was necessary. Their assessment of the risks, benefits, and need to operate varied widely.[3] Because of this, we encourage you to cross-reference your doctor's recommendation with your own online research. Look for details on the particular circumstances where surgery is recommended, and consider looking at the treatment guidelines discussed in chapter 5. In some cases, such as a hernia, surgery is often the mainstay of treatment. In other cases, such as back pain, nonsurgical options may work just as well. Keep in mind the importance of trustworthy websites and the potential pitfalls of nonauthoritative sites like Facebook and Reddit.

Understanding more about your condition and asking questions before making decisions about surgery significantly increases the likelihood of reaching an informed decision.[4] If, after talking with your doctors and doing your own research, you have any doubt or hesitation about your decision, consider a second opinion. Research suggests that nonsurgeons are more likely to incorporate patient preferences in their decision-making, so consider seeking a second opinion from a nonsurgeon who is highly knowledgeable and skilled in the field. If you're considering surgery on a heart valve, for example, you may be better off seeking a second opinion from a cardiologist rather than a cardiothoracic surgeon.

Choosing Your Surgeon

If you decide that surgery is the right option, your referring doctor will often recommend a surgeon or surgical center for your procedure. Sometimes, the choice of surgeon is left entirely up to the patient, who may be limited to some degree by their health insurance and its list of viable in-network doctors. No matter the case, it's important to do research on your surgeon's track record. Anytime you go under the knife, even for a minor procedure, you put yourself at risk for life-threatening complications like the one Leah experienced. Research shows, as anyone might expect, that some doctors have better track records than others when it comes to complications.[5]

There are a number of online tools available to help you figure out how your surgeon ranks. ProPublica created an online surgeon scorecard that provides information on more than 16,000 surgeons across the United States.[6] The nonprofit Consumers' Checkbook/Center for the Study of Services also put together a similar rating system for surgeons. Their site includes an analysis of more than 4 million operations conducted by 50,000 surgeons in the United States.[7]

If data are not available for your surgeon, then see if you can find out how many procedures the hospital does per year. You may even be able to find complication rates and compare how hospitals perform on sites from Medicare and The Leapfrog Group.[8,9] It can help to find a center that has done the procedure many times since the research suggests that this is correlated with better outcomes.[10] This is because, generally speaking, the more times a center does a procedure, the better they become. Also, the medical team develops experience with a wide range of complications and variations. In some cases, you may have been recommended a very unique surgery that has not been widely practiced. In this case, consider going to a tertiary care center, which is a large hospital that provides highly specialized care. While they may not do as many of the "routine" cases, they are often highly experienced in the unique cases.

If you're still not sure about the surgeon you've selected, even after all your online research, it's worth trying to schedule a meeting to discuss your case with them directly. Meeting them in person may give you a better sense of whether they are the right fit for you and your particular case.

In addition to the surgeon, it's important to be knowledgeable about the team administering the anesthesia. Oftentimes, you will have an appointment with someone from the anesthesia team before your surgery. If not, you should proactively ask to set it up. There are questions you can ask that will help you understand the type of anesthesia you will be getting and what to expect. We've included these questions at the end of this chapter. Inform the anesthesiologist of any prior bad experiences you've had with anesthetic as well as your medical history. Depending on your insurance, and where the procedure is scheduled, you may have a limited say in who performs the anesthesia. If you don't feel comfortable after speaking with them, ask your surgeon or staff at the surgical center about other options.

Preparing for Surgery

Studies suggest that there are things you can do prior to surgery to improve your health outcomes and relieve some of the administrative and logistical stress that might accompany your procedure.

Call your insurance company to avoid any surprise medical bills. Ask your doctor's office the exact CPT code for the procedure, the associated diagnosis, and its ICD code. Then call your insurance company, give them the name of your doctors, where the surgery will take place, and the list of codes to understand how much of the bill the insurance company will cover and how much you might need to pay out of pocket. It might also be worth asking them about what coverage you have for rehabilitation after surgery since it can help inform those decisions.

Connect with close friends and family to let them know about your procedure. In all likelihood, your surgery will go smoothly, but it's always good to be prepared. Create a list of contacts and let them know where your surgery is taking place, your doctor's name and number, how long your recovery is expected to be, and what they can do in the event of a complication. You may ask one or two key people to connect with each other so that they can work together to help organize meal deliveries or other forms of support.

Ask your doctor about changes you can make to improve your outcome. For some surgeries, increasing physical activity or cutting back on smoking, drinking, or other health-harming behaviors prior to the procedure can make an important difference to the outcome of your surgery. Your doctor may also want you to get any chronic diseases under control before going in for surgery. For example, if you have hypertension, your blood pressure should be controlled. Generally speaking, doctors avoid doing an elective procedure when a chronic disease is uncontrolled since it could make the situation worse.

Determine how to manage your pain. Almost all surgeries result in pain, which needs to be managed. The opioid crisis in the

United States has made many people wary of accepting this type of pain medication. While it is important to be cautious, opioids should still be considered as part of your pain management plan, alongside other options ranging from over-the-counter painkillers to nondrug approaches. Work with your medical team to put together a plan and find the right combination for your needs. It is important to figure out a regimen that works for you while you are still in the hospital so that your pain is adequately controlled when you get home. If not, there is a risk that you may be in more pain than is acceptable to you when you get home.

Prepare for your recovery. After your surgery, you'll likely be tired and have less energy for daily activities, such as preparing meals or cleaning your house. To avoid becoming overwhelmed, try to prepare a few days' worth of meals in advance, set out loose clothing that will be comfortable to wear given where your incisions will be, and try to purchase any bandages or lotions and fill any prescriptions that you may need in advance. Think through the logistics of your life in the days after surgery. If your bathroom and bedroom are on separate floors, it might be worth looking into a bedside commode to minimize trips up and down the stairs. A doctor may even be able to prescribe one so that it is covered by insurance. If you are undergoing a major procedure or are frail to begin with, see if your doctor can order a home safety assessment to help reduce your risk of falls.[11]

The Day of Surgery

On the day of surgery, you should have instructions from the health care team on what to wear (often loose-fitting clothes, no jewelry), eat (usually no food prior to the procedure), and where to go. You should also have instructions on what to do with your usual medications as well as any additional ones you might need to take.

One of the most important things that you can do on the day of your surgery is to bring along someone who understands your wishes and is willing to act as your health care power of attorney, meaning that they can make health decisions on your behalf if you are not able to. We encourage you to read through chapter 10 to learn more about how to choose your health proxy and the discussions to have with your proxy before you go for surgery.

Having a companion with you is also useful for any discussions that you have with your surgical or medical team after the procedure, when the effects of the anesthesia have not yet worn off. If you want more details on the procedure itself, you can also ask the hospital or surgical center for the operative note that describes what took place during the surgery. An operative note is often dictated right after a surgical procedure, and it becomes a part of your medical record. It can be useful to know what was done to help you convey the information to other members of the health care team that you meet during your recovery and beyond.

Managing Your Recovery

The post-surgery recovery period can be divided into two phases: the first phase in the hospital and the second phase at home.

Recovering in the Hospital

In the hospital, the main challenge is keeping track of all the information that the nurses and doctors will share with you. Similar to our recommendations in other chapters, it can be helpful to write down what you are told and ask any questions you may have. Make sure you understand everything that is going on, and don't be afraid to ask the nurses if you don't. There are many different medical teams and providers in the hospital, and they may not always be aware of what the other is doing or recommending. You can help reduce miscommunication and medical errors by being proactive, making sure you understand what each team is recommending, and keeping track of what is being done. You may consider having a health advocate or companion help you during this critical phase given the pain and discomfort you might be facing.

One very basic thing you can do as you recover in the hospital is to remind any health care provider that comes into the room to wash their hands. Research shows that even though handwashing—with hand sanitizer or soap and water—can reduce infections in the hospital, staff sometimes skip this important step.[12] Studies have shown the benefits of patients helping to promote good hand hygiene, though they also recognize the awkwardness of asking a health care professional to wash their hands.[13] If possible, try framing a handwashing request in a neutral, collaborative way, such as "I'm really concerned about getting an infection. Would you mind washing your hands once more to help ease my anxiety?"

Before you're discharged from the hospital, be sure to explore some key questions with the relevant members of your medical team:

- Should I continue to take pain medication and, if so, how frequently?

- Should I be on the lookout for any symptoms that may indicate an important health problem?

- Will I be responsible for drains or dressing changes and, if so, how frequently?

- How much exercise and activity should I do, and when? Studies show that getting moving sooner helps reduce complications. You may want to ask about meeting with a physical therapist.

- Are there any deep breathing exercises I can do? Some deep breathing exercises can help reduce your risk of pneumonia after surgery.

You might also consider asking for a copy of your medical records, which are different from the paperwork handed out at discharge. Your records are the medical notes detailing your hospital stay. These notes are more technical and can be invaluable during follow-up visits, especially for doctors who were not involved in your care in the hospital.

Recovering at Home

The transition back home is a challenging stage. If it doesn't go smoothly, you may end up having to head back to the hospital to manage any complications. There are a few things you need to consider during your recovery at home, including your activity level, your medications, caring for any wounds or incisions from surgery, and managing your emotions. The specifics for each of these elements of your recovery will be unique to your situation and should be discussed in detail with the doctors and nurses at the hospital before you go home.

Once you're back home, your job is to make sure that you understand the state of your condition and that you're doing your best to follow your medical team's guidance for recovery. Many people find that it's easier to keep track of things on a simple chart. In addition to tracking your medications, it's also important to track any persistent or new symptoms since they may be a sign of a complication. We've included a sample recovery tracker at the end of this chapter. Apps to track your recovery, such as SeamlessMD, are becoming increasingly common, and your hospital may even have their own system that you can sign in to.

In addition to tracking your physical recovery, you should also be aware of how you're feeling emotionally. It's easy to start feeling isolated and alone as you recover. Even if you're surrounded by caring friends or family, you may still feel as though no one understands what you're going through. Depending on the type of surgery you've had, you may also struggle with how the procedure has changed the way your body looks or moves. These aren't easy issues to deal with. The section in chapter 8 about social support may be useful to help you deal with some of these challenges.

A full physical and emotional recovery often takes longer than a medical recovery. To the extent that you can, take things slow and try not to put pressure on yourself to speed up the pace of your recovery.

Tools to Help Manage Your Surgery and Recovery

Worksheet: Best-Case/Worst-Case Scenarios

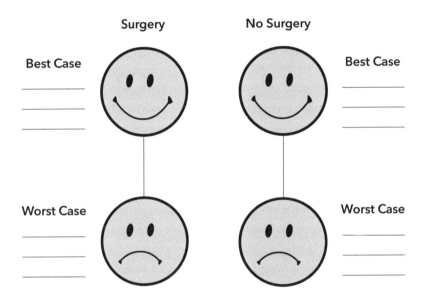

Adapted from Kruser JM, Taylor LJ, Campbell TC, et al. "Best case/worst case": training surgeons to use a novel communication tool for high-risk acute surgical problems. *Journal of Pain and Symptom Management.* 2017;53(4):711–719.e5.

Questions to Ask the Anesthesia Team

What type of anesthesia will I get?

Options include local anesthesia that numbs the area, sedation (also referred to as twilight sleep), epidural (often used in labor), and general anesthesia. Your doctor should be able to go over the details of the type of anesthesia that you will receive.

Am I at risk for complications from anesthesia?

Ask if there are things that put you at higher risk for complications from the anesthesia. Ask what (if anything) can be done to minimize your risks. You should take these risks into account when weighing the decision to undergo surgery.

What can I expect when I wake up?

The doctor should be able to give you a sense of how you will feel when you wake up. They can inform you about what they will do to control pain, nausea, and other symptoms.

What are my options for pain control?

Try to understand all the options available, which can include opiates, nonopiates, as well as nondrug alternatives. Your doctor can advise you on how to weigh the risks and benefits of these different options as well as address any concerns you might have. For example, given the current opioid crisis, many people worry about getting addicted to pain medications. The doctor can discuss these concerns and how to minimize the risk.

What should I do to prepare for the procedure?

Make sure you understand all the pre-surgery instructions, like when to stop eating, whether or not to take your regular medications, and what to wear to the hospital. These can make a big difference on the day of the procedure.

Post-Surgery Recovery Tracker

	Day 1	Day 2	Day 3	Day 4	Day 5	Day 6	Day 7
Pain (rate on a 10-point scale)							
Bleeding (minimal, moderate, significant)							
Wound (note changes in color and discharge)							
Appetite (poor, good, great)							
New symptoms							
Walking (minutes per day)							
Bowel movement (number of times per day and consistency)							
Urination (number of times per day)							
Pain medication (record the amount you take to track how much you need and the trend over time)							
Morning medication							
Afternoon medication							
Evening medication							

Red flag symptoms _____

Follow-up appointment _____

8 | Lifestyle Treatment Options

For some people, the recommended treatment is neither surgical nor drug related. Take Morris Jackson, a thirty-seven-year-old man with a busy work life and an even busier personal life as a husband and father of two girls under the age of five.* Mo thought of himself as relatively healthy and was surprised when he randomly checked his blood pressure at a grocery store kiosk one day and it was elevated. But, then again, he was at the store with his kids and figured that was enough to get anyone's blood pressure up.

The next day, during his lunch break, Mo went to the pharmacy to check his blood pressure again, assuming that he'd get a more accurate reading at a calmer time, but his levels were still too high. Like many of us when life gets busy, Mo had missed his routine checkups over the last couple of years. But with two troubling blood pressure results, he thought it was worthwhile to finally book his annual checkup and talk to his doctor about what the readings might mean. Still, he wasn't particularly worried.

After dropping his kids off at daycare one morning, Mo went to his doctor's office for his appointment. The nurse doing intake took his blood pressure and let out a murmur at the unexpected

---

* Name has been changed to protect privacy.

reading. She repeated the measurement to be sure it was correct and then told Mo that the doctor would meet with him to go over what it meant. As Mo waited, he thought about what might be causing his high blood pressure. Perhaps he hadn't really recognized how much stress he was under. Or maybe it was just a result of all the rich meals he'd been eating and the free cookies he was always sneaking at the office. He should definitely lay off the cookies, he thought.

The doctor went through what seemed like an endless series of questions and examined him. She told him that the blood pressure readings at the store and pharmacy and now in the office suggested that he might have high blood pressure, or hypertension, but she wanted to run some tests to be sure. Could he go to the lab today and come back in a week for a follow-up visit? "Absolutely," replied Mo, making a mental note to ask his wife to pick up the kids that day. He booked a follow-up appointment for the next week and left the office.

The week flew by, and Mo had little time to dwell on his health. With the exception of one quick search online about high blood pressure, he hadn't really given it much thought. Before he knew it, Mo was sitting across from the doctor again, waiting to hear about his test results. He noticed the slight hesitation as she prepared to speak, and he thought, "That's not a good sign." His intuition was right—the doctor informed Mo that he had hypertension and diabetes. His blood tests showed that his average blood sugar over the last few months was around 300 mg/dL, about twice what it should be. As the words sunk in, Mo felt a rising panic. Would he need insulin? Were his kids at risk? Was he going to have a heart attack? The questions swirled in his head even as the doctor continued with her explanation.

Mo tried hard to focus on her words. The first step, she said, would be a series of lifestyle changes. He would have to reduce the sugar and salt in his diet and see a nutritionist. He would need to get more exercise. They would try this for three months and then repeat the blood tests. If his blood pressure and sugar levels were still too high, Mo would need medications. This often happened, she cautioned him, but it was worth checking to see what impact diet and exercise had. The doctor tried to reassure Mo that there were many options to treat his condition, but it was a matter of taking it one step at a time. With that, the appointment was over, and Mo left the office feeling overwhelmed.

The Impact of Lifestyle on Health

Lifestyle factors such as poor diet, smoking, and lack of physical activity play a major role in causing some of the most prevalent diseases in the world, including type 2 diabetes, hypertension, and heart disease.[1] These diseases account for most of the deaths around the world, more deaths than due to all infectious diseases combined.[2]

Many of us think of lifestyle changes as an opportunity to prevent disease. We stop smoking because we want to reduce our chance of lung cancer, or we exercise to keep our hearts healthy. While this is certainly an important approach, it overlooks the value of lifestyle changes to treat health conditions that are already present.

For some conditions, like appendicitis, a lifestyle change will not play a role in treatment. But, in many cases, the best type of treatment isn't a medication or a surgical procedure but a lifestyle change. For people recovering from a heart attack, for example, exercise counseling and training have been shown to save lives.[3] In people with peripheral arterial disease—blockages in the blood vessels of the legs—an exercise program can be more beneficial than a stent (a metal or plastic tube used to keep a blood vessel open).[4] With lifestyle changes, the side effects that drugs or a surgical procedure might bring can be avoided.

Despite the benefits, some doctors still hesitate to include lifestyle changes as part of their ideal treatment. Doctors, as we've described throughout this book, tend to advocate for science-based approaches whenever possible. However, this can be challenging with lifestyle changes. Many of the research studies on the impact of lifestyle changes on health only include a small number of participants or were only done for a short period of time. Some of them are observational studies, which can suggest that two things are linked (for example, eating a certain diet and heart attacks) but cannot confirm cause and effect.

Other times, there is evidence of benefit, but doctors don't have the training, time, or appropriate incentives to offer effective counseling on lifestyle changes. A good example of this is quitting smoking. Experts recommend that doctors use the five A's strategy:

1. **Ask** about tobacco use.
2. **Advise** patients to quit using tobacco.
3. **Assess** if the patient is willing to stop.
4. **Assist** using counseling, nicotine replacement, and medications.
5. **Arrange** follow-up contact, ideally within a week of the quit date.

While this is a thoughtful approach, studies suggest that many doctors don't go into all these details, perhaps because they just don't have the time.[5] This means that the onus is often on the patient to figure out which lifestyle changes can help their condition. Research suggests that people are increasingly going online to figure this out.[6] This chapter offers some suggestions to help you find the information you need to figure out which lifestyle changes make sense for you.

Doctor-Recommended Lifestyle Changes

Most of us think of exercise and nutrition when we think of lifestyle changes, but the concept is much broader than that. Almost all lifestyle choices fit into six broad categories:

1. **Nutrition:** what you eat and drink and how often

2. **Physical activity:** the type of exercises you do and their frequency, along with other forms of physical therapy that can help your body recover

3. **Tobacco and other drugs:** tobacco, caffeine, alcohol, and recreational drugs that may have an important impact on your health

4. **Environmental factors:** both negative and positive factors, ranging from pollution and allergens to safety grab bars to prevent falls

5. **Mental health and wellness:** your happiness level, the amount of sleep you get, and how you deal with stress

6. **Social support and caregivers:** level of support from friends, caregivers, or others with the same condition as you

If your doctor recommends a lifestyle change as part of your treatment, make sure that you understand what changes they think would be most useful. For example, if you have high blood pressure, your doctor might recommend that you change your diet. But you need to be sure you understand what specific changes to your diet would be most beneficial for your condition. It's likely that your doctor would recommend the DASH diet, which stands for Dietary Approaches to Stop Hypertension. This diet has been rigorously tested in randomized controlled trials and shown to lower blood pressure and reduce the risk of a heart attack.[7,8]

When you leave your doctor's office, head home and do your own research on the recommendation. In this case, where your doctor has been specific about the recommendation, look up the DASH diet rather than a more generic search like "What should I eat to lower my blood pressure?" Try to understand the key principles underlying the diet and figure out how you can apply them to your life. You might find the experiences of others useful as you think through how to cut back on some foods or how to make your new lifestyle changes stick.

Sometimes, online resources will be complemented by offline ones like helplines or in-person events. Speaking one-on-one with an expert can get you advice that is tailored to your situation. Consider giving your health insurance company a call as well. There are likely to be benefits, often required by law,[9] that you can take advantage of. If your insurance company doesn't offer the benefits you need, but you still want to find a way to pay for items related to your change in lifestyle, explore the possibility of a Flexible Spending Account or Health Savings Account, which can often be used if you have a letter from your doctor. Doing the research may help you reduce the financial burden as you work to improve your health.

Exploring Lifestyle Changes on Your Own

Let's say that your doctor doesn't recommend any lifestyle-based options to treat your condition. It's still worthwhile for you to explore lifestyle changes on your own. Often there are lifestyle changes that can complement the other treatments your doctor recommends. For example, suppose you need surgery to remove your gallbladder. Research shows that stopping smoking before the procedure can significantly cut complication rates.[10] Another study found that exercise programs before surgery (called prehabilitation) can also improve some outcomes.[11]

If you're searching online for lifestyle changes that can help you treat or manage your condition, apply the same tools we talked about in earlier chapters when approaching an online search. For example, if you've been diagnosed with gout, you'd want to start with a more general search like "lifestyle changes for gout" instead of something more specific like "diet to treat gout." If your general search leads you to diet as an option, then you can explore that in more detail. Refer back to our guidance on trustworthy websites in chapter 2 as you work through the process. To avoid untested or unreliable approaches, consider adding a search on the scientific recommendations for whatever lifestyle-based approach you're considering, such as "scientific guidelines on gout diet."

Also keep in mind the adage "first do no harm." If the recommendation is to stop all medications and replace them with a new diet, it's important to think about the potential harm such a move might have. There are far too many stories of people hurting themselves or their loved ones in an effort to find a cure for their condition. In many Facebook groups for parents of children with autism, for example, people post about the curative benefits of adding bleach and acidic juice to their children's drinks to rid them of the disease. At least one hundred cases of this have been reported to Child Protective Services since 2016.[12] While it's tempting to think that this could never happen to us, it isn't hard to fall into this trap when you're looking for ways to treat a distressing health condition.

Once you find a credible set of options that you are considering pursuing, book a follow-up visit with your doctor to discuss the approach with them. Try asking questions in a way that gives your doctor the opportunity to raise concerns and be a part of your decision-making process. For example, you might say something like, "Do you think there is any harm in trying the Mediterranean diet for a month to see if it lowers my blood sugar?" instead of "I think I'm going to try a Mediterranean diet for a while and see how that affects my blood sugar." You might also ask, "Are there other lifestyle options I should consider?" to further engage your doctor in your research.

One thing you may want to ask about specifically is whether there are any specialists you should see or programs that you qualify for. For example, a nutritionist might be helpful if you're planning to make changes to your diet. An occupational therapist could help with advice on how to manage your daily activities. There may also be specific programs you can enroll in that may offer supervised lifestyle treatment options and advice. For example, the Centers for Disease Control and Prevention (CDC) has a list of providers that offer lifestyle programs for diabetes.[13]

If, in speaking with your doctor, you find that they are overly dismissive or discouraging of your approach, consider getting a second opinion. As discussed in chapter 4, getting a second opinion is a perfectly acceptable practice. If you want to speak specifically about lifestyle changes, consider seeing an integrative medicine specialist since they will be knowledgeable about other nondrug forms of treatment. Through them, you may find even more lifestyle treatment options for you to consider, or you may learn that there isn't a major role for lifestyle changes in your treatment plan.

Mental Health

It can be easy to overlook the importance of mental health when it comes to physical illness, but there are definite links between the two. For example, 20 percent to 40 percent of people report depression after a heart attack.[14] To the extent that you can, be proactive about how you approach your mental health after being diagnosed with a serious condition. Search online to see if others with your condition have noticed any feelings of depression, isolation, or other mental health issues. Consider joining support groups—online or in person—to help you feel less isolated and to connect you with others who are going through a similar situation.

It's also important to consider how your online searches about your condition may be affecting your mental health. *Cyberchondria* is a growing concern among many health care practitioners as more and more patients report anxiety and stress related to their online searches about their symptoms and real or imagined conditions. It can be hard to distinguish between valid concerns and needless anxiety, and even experts can get thrown off when dealing with their own illnesses.[15]

To help you navigate these issues, be sure to bring up any mental health concerns with your doctor. Studies show that it often takes years after the start of symptoms for people to get a diagnosis of a mental health disorder,[16] so you're better off letting your doctor know early on how you're feeling. They can help direct you to additional mental health support if needed.

Social Support

The support of friends, family, and others is an important aspect to consider as it relates to your health. Studies have shown that a person's level of social support and integration has a great effect on health outcomes for particular conditions.[17] Much like your mental health, it pays to be proactive when it comes to your social support network.

There are a number of apps that can help you stay connected to your existing network of family and friends. Many of these apps help people update loved ones and acquaintances on new health developments and notify their social network if they're in need of help, whether that be a home-cooked meal or a drive to the hospital. The internet now provides new avenues to expand a person's social support network substantially through forums, blogs, and social media platforms. While there is a risk of misinformation on these unregulated and often unsupervised platforms, they do bring many benefits.

Rachelle Downton, who we introduced in chapter 1, spoke to us about how important social media networks were to her during her son's illness and throughout his recovery. After Xavier had been admitted to the hospital, and before doctors were able to diagnose him with AFM, his condition worsened. His skin hurt so much that he couldn't bear to be touched or even have clothes or sheets covering him. By then, he was completely paralyzed and having trouble with his breathing. In the moment, Rachelle wasn't ready to reach out, but once Xavier was diagnosed and had a treatment plan in place, Rachelle joined groups such as the UK Transverse Myelitis Society Facebook group and other similar American and Canadian networks. "I wasn't participating in the discussion at first because there was just so much going on," Rachelle said. "But it was good even in that moment to read about other parents' experiences and know there was support. It was actually later though that those groups became even more important. That's where we learned about long-term consequences and what Xavier's recovery might look like a year or two down the road. It's also where we learned what to expect from the system itself, things like what the school board could offer or other occupational therapy benefits that the government offered."

Dr. Riley Bove, a neurologist at the University of California, San Francisco, whose son was also diagnosed with AFM, had a similar experience. Though her neurology training and her position offered some advantages—as she put it, her son had access to "immediate diagnosis, hospitalization, and the kitchen sink of available medications"—she was still anxious about her son's recovery and joined a Facebook support group for help. "Through the Facebook group, I learned about recommended rehabilitation experts, electrical stimulation devices and settings, and templates for letters to insurers," she wrote in a recent *New England Journal of Medicine* article.[18] "When my son began to protest against constant therapy appointments. . .other parents provided a number of effective (and endearing) ways of coaxing their child to persist with exercises."

The benefits of support groups also flow back to the medical community. Through her online networks, Rachelle was able to connect to researchers who were trying to determine the cause of AFM. She sent some of Xavier's specimens to the researchers to help with their work. Parents who have shared their experiences via the Facebook group have also become part of working groups on AFM led by clinicians.

In addition to these personal anecdotes, the scientific literature supports the idea that adding online communities to your existing social support network can be beneficial, so we encourage you to consider it. A systematic review found that people get emotional support, learn new information, and feel more empowered through their use of social media. They also have an opportunity to express their emotions and compare the symptoms of their condition to others. This can reduce the isolation and loneliness that often come with having a disease. On the whole, people felt more confident in talking to their doctors and managing their condition.[19]

Sticking With It

Engaging in lifestyle changes and becoming empowered takes a lot of effort, but the impact can be quite profound. For Mo, whose story started this chapter, his path wasn't easy, but it was transformative. Once he got over the shock of his diagnosis, he was determined to do everything he could to get better: he changed his diet, exercised more often, and started tracking his blood pressure and blood sugar. He learned to manage food-related social situations like birthday parties and dinners out with friends without appearing rude. The times that he relaxed his diet or failed to exercise were soon reflected in his blood pressure and blood sugar levels, which would motivate him to get back on track. The results of all his efforts were evident when he went for his follow-up appointment about six months after his diagnosis. His blood sugar and blood pressure were completely normal. We should note here that this is quite remarkable. With no medications at all, Mo had managed to control his diabetes and hypertension. While we recognize that not everyone will have these kinds of results, we are hopeful that you can find ways to make lifestyle changes that are meaningful for your health.

9 | Complementary and Alternative Treatments

The driving force behind this book is a desire to ensure people have access to the most relevant and credible health information available. Unfortunately, this is a particular challenge when it comes to alternative treatments because, for the most part, there isn't enough reliable research on the impact and side effects of these approaches.

Alternative treatments replace conventional medical treatments, whereas complementary treatments are used in addition to a conventional medical treatment.[1] These alternative and complementary treatments can range from dietary supplements and herbal remedies to mind-body techniques such as acupuncture and yoga, as well as ancient healing systems such as Ayurveda and traditional Chinese medicine. These types of treatments are popular worldwide[2] and have existed, in some cases, for centuries. Despite this, there continues to be a significant lack of evidence backing many of these treatments.

Part of the challenge is due to the availability of funding. A pharmaceutical company may invest millions of research dollars in a conventional medication to treat migraines, for example, with the plan to earn that money back in sales of a patented drug. It would be a challenge to find a company willing to invest the same amount of money in something like meditation, which lacks the same profit-making potential.

Another reason is that, historically, the health care community has been focused on finding treatments or cures for acute diseases, such as pneumonia, HIV/AIDS, tuberculosis, and cholera. These illnesses are better suited to treatment and prevention through conventional medicine, which is why researchers focused their efforts in that area. In the past few decades however, chronic conditions such as diabetes, heart disease, and arthritis have become the leading causes of death and disability.

Since complementary and alternative treatments may potentially have a greater impact on chronic conditions than on acute diseases, there is now a rising interest throughout the scientific community to better understand complementary and alternative medicine and to apply the same scientific rigor to investigate the potential benefits and side effects of these treatments. But there is still not enough research on many of these approaches.

In the absence of solid research, many people choose to pursue alternative or complementary therapies because of word of mouth or anecdotal evidence, much of which they find online. Others believe that alternative medicines are somehow more natural, and therefore better, than conventional medicines, perhaps also assuming that more natural approaches will have fewer side effects. But that thinking can sometimes lead you down a dangerous path.

Potential Pitfalls of Complementary and Alternative Treatments

Take the case of red yeast rice. For years, alternative medicine practitioners have been touting the benefits of using extracts from rice fermented using a specific type of red yeast. The extract sometimes naturally contains a compound called monacolin K, which is identical to the active ingredient used in some statin drugs.[3]

On websites and in online forums, hundreds of people have claimed that the extract has helped them reduce their cholesterol without any side effects. Many folks on these sites offer a fair take on the benefits of the extract while also highlighting the potential pitfalls, namely that the red yeast rice extracts on the market are unregulated and may contain either too little or too much monacolin K. The best alternative treatment sites also warn that too much monacolin K could lead to health issues, and they uniformly recommend a conversation with a doctor before taking the supplement.

But other websites present a more one-sided point of view. Take the website run by Dr. Sam Robbins, who is not a medical doctor but has a PhD in molecular and medical pharmacology. He says that red yeast rice has been used daily in Asia for centuries with "no problems whatsoever."[4] This is a broad and sweeping statement that can't, by the sheer vastness of the claim, be based on hard evidence—there is simply no way to document every single use of red yeast rice extract in Asia over centuries and be sure that there has never been a side effect.

What happens when people read websites like the one by Sam Robbins and take the information as absolute truth? For some, they end up like JS, the unnamed subject of a peer-reviewed medical article.[5] JS was a relatively healthy sixty-four-year-old woman who was surprised to find, on a routine visit with her doctor, that her cholesterol was too high. Her doctor recommended statins, but she wanted to weigh her options. In doing her research, she came across red yeast rice as an alternative method of lowering cholesterol, and she ordered some from NOW Foods, a popular natural supplement store.

JS began taking about 1,200 mg of red yeast extract every day. About a month later, she noticed she was more tired than usual and didn't have the appetite she used to have. She didn't think much of it until later, when her urine and stools started changing color and she noticed the whites of her eyes had turned yellow. Eventually, she was diagnosed with acute liver injury. She was transferred to a specialized hospital where further testing revealed that her liver had been damaged by the red yeast rice supplement and her recovery would take months.

JS is not alone in her story. There are several case reports of liver injury from red yeast rice that have been recorded in the literature.[6] Because of the lack of regulation of natural health products and alternative supplements, there was no way for JS to know how much monacolin K was in any given container. In the end, her injuries were a result of an overdose of this naturally occurring drug.

Potential Benefits of Complementary and Alternative Treatments

While the potential damage complementary and alternative medicines can do to the body can be severe, there may be significant benefits to these approaches that also can't be overlooked. Some of the most successful conventional medicines available today have their roots in alternative therapies. For example, one of the most effective antimalarial medications—artemether—is derived from artemisinin, which is used in traditional Chinese medicine.[7] Initially met with skepticism and resistance, the treatment has now become firmly established. The scientist who discovered artemisinin was one of the recipients of the 2015 Nobel Prize in Physiology or Medicine.

In order to better understand the potential benefits and risks of complementary and alternative medicines, the US government created the National Center for Complementary and Integrative Health (NCCIH). The mission of the NCCIH is to define, through rigorous scientific investigation, the usefulness and safety of complementary and integrative health interventions and their roles in improving health and health care.

If you are considering an alternative treatment approach, the NCCIH website (https://www.nccih.nih.gov/) is a great place to start your research. The site provides summaries of recent studies supported by the institution that are written in plain, nontechnical language. If you don't find the answers you need on the NCCIH website, you can also look at sites such as PubMed or Google Scholar to find additional research. The papers that appear on these websites will likely be more technical, but the abstract (summary) for each study will give you some clues as to the major findings.[8]

In addition to looking for scientific papers, it's worth looking into expert opinions on the treatment. One option is to speak with your pharmacist, who can offer their opinion on the treatment and also explore how the treatment might interact with any other medications you are taking. You can also consider signing up for a professional medical resource such as UpToDate (https://www.uptodate .com/home) or DynaMed (https://www.dynamed.com/). While geared toward doctors, sites like these can be helpful to you too. It might be worth checking with a librarian at your hospital library to help you access these and other resources to find more authoritative information.

If your online searches for scientific papers or expert opinions take you to personal stories from people who have experience with the treatment, take their opinions into consideration, but make sure that you are balancing those opinions with your own follow-up research. For example, if you read a number of stories about the benefits people have experienced with a particular treatment, be sure to do your due diligence and specifically search for side effects or risks related to the treatment as well. In addition to the guidance offered in chapter 2 on trustworthy websites, we encourage you to be especially cautious of any website that is trying to sell or promote their alternative treatment products or services.

One thing to keep in mind as you read through personal stories is the influence of the placebo and nocebo effects described in chapter 6.

Studies show that alternative practitioners are sometimes better than conventional health care providers at connecting with patients.[9] Because of this, people may walk away from a visit with an alternative practitioner with a better understanding of the benefits of alternative medicines than of conventional medicines, and their online posts may reflect more of a placebo effect.

No Matter What, Talk to Your Doctor

If you're considering the use of complementary or alternative medicines, we strongly recommend that you speak with your doctor after you have done your research. Many of us hesitate to bring up these approaches with our primary care doctors,[10] perhaps because we're unsure whether our doctor will support an alternative approach. Still, it's important to at least try to discuss it with your doctor so that they can raise any immediate concerns they might have.

A neutral way to bring the topic up is to say something like, "Would it hurt for me to try this other type of alternative treatment first, before pursuing the course of treatment you recommend?" Or, you could ask whether you could pursue both treatment options at the same time: "Would there be anything wrong with me trying a complementary treatment while I pursue the course of action you recommend?"

You might also want to review the research you've done on the alternative approach with your doctor, or at least give them some indication of how you determined that an alternative treatment might work for you. This may provide the doctor additional context around your thinking and creates an opportunity for shared decision-making.

If your doctor isn't open to speaking to you in detail about the alternative approach, consider seeking out an integrative medicine consult, either in person or online from a reputable provider. Integrative medicine practitioners walk the line between conventional medicine and alternative medicine. There are some online resources, such as the Andrew Weil Center for Integrative Medicine at The University of Arizona, that can help you find a practitioner in your city or state. If you cannot find one locally, institutions such as the Cleveland Clinic offer virtual visits.

Choosing an Alternative Care Practitioner

Just like a search for any type of health care provider, you will need to do careful research before deciding on a complementary, alternative, or integrative medicine practitioner. Look into the practitioner's qualifications, years of experience, and patient testimonials. To the extent possible, make sure that their claims are credible and any degrees or certificates come from reputable institutions. Keep in mind that verifying these claims will be difficult for the same reason that verifying the efficacy of complementary and alternative treatments is difficult—there is currently a lack of regulation and standardized qualifications across the field.

Generally speaking, each of your providers should be open to the idea of you receiving advice from another practitioner, even if they don't always agree with the advice offered. For example, your doctor may have a concern about an alternative treatment. Or your naturopath may feel that your doctor's recommendations are too extreme. Both of these situations are completely within the norm. But be cautious about any practitioner who delivers blanket statements like, "I don't ever believe in surgery for this condition" or "I don't think you can trust the treatment they give in hospitals." That may be a sign that your provider is not open to any other approaches, even ones that are backed by credible evidence.

Going to two or three different alternative medicine practitioners can be a good option even if you like the first one you speak with. It will help you walk away with a strong understanding of the variety of options that exist. Whenever you can, use the internet to double-check any advice or recommendations your practitioner gives you before deciding to follow their course of treatment.

You may also want to speak to your practitioner about costs. Complementary and alternative therapies can be costly. By some estimates, about $30 billion is spent every year in the United States on such treatments.[11] Your insurance company may cover the cost of your consultation as a specialist visit but may not cover all the treatments an integrative medicine provider may recommend. Some insurance companies may not even cover the cost of the initial consultation. If this is the case, ask the practitioner if they know of any ways to reduce your out-of-pocket costs. As integrative medicine is an emerging field, many practitioners will have had people come into their office with similar concerns regarding payment; it is likely that they have worthwhile guidance for you on the financial front.

Coordinating Your Care

In general, when you decide to incorporate complementary or alternative medicines into your treatment plan, you'll end up doing more research and work to make sure that you're managing your care properly. In an ideal situation, all your care providers would share information with each other directly, with your complementary practitioner checking in with your regular doctor first before suggesting any new medicine or treatment. In practice, you will likely be the one in charge of coordinating your own care and will need to be comfortable being the go-between.

One way to do this effectively is to track the information in your medical history form, which we described in detail in chapter 2. At the beginning of each appointment with either your conventional or alternative care provider, let them know that you would like to update them on the treatments you're receiving from your other care provider. Track any medications and supplements you plan to take, along with the dosage and, in the case of vitamins or other alternative supplements, the brand of the product. (Since many alternative medications are considered supplements by the FDA, they do not face the same level of scrutiny as conventional medications, so you should be aware of the possibility of adulteration, which means that the supplement contains something not stated on the label.) Your conventional and complementary care providers can let you know of any medication contraindications that they are aware of. They may also be able to give you guidance on dosing since inconsistent dosing of a conventional medicine and some alternative medicines can lead to side effects or lack of efficacy. Keep track of your symptoms so that you have a more detailed idea of what might be working or not.

Overcoming the Challenges

Navigating your way down the complementary and alternative medicine path will not be easy, but it could have major benefits. Ben Hunter was in his mid-fifties when he was diagnosed with prostate cancer.[12] Fortunately, the cancer hadn't metastasized and it was slow growing. This meant that Ben had time to choose from a variety of options that his doctors suggested: radical prostatectomy, traditional radiation therapy, radioactive seeds, freezing the prostate, or burning the prostate. All are conventional courses of treatment, with a wide variety of studies to back up their efficacy.

"At the time, what most hit me were the side effects of treatment," Ben said in an interview with the Harvard Health Blog. "The doctors told me that with surgery there was a 30% chance of impotence, and maybe a 5% chance of incontinence. That's a pretty stunning thing to hear, when you consider yourself in the prime of life and healthy. But radiation wasn't any better. It had similar complications, with slightly different percentages, but it might also cause rectal damage. So I continued to research the various options and compare the numbers."

With the help of his wife, who did occasional research on medical conditions for her friends, Ben decided to research other options online. "From my research, I knew that in Japan, prostate cancer was very rare," Ben said. "But when Japanese men move to America, after a generation or two, their prostate cancer rates are the same as American men. So this led me to hypothesize that prostate cancer is a lifestyle disease."

So, Ben started to make a series of lifestyle changes. He ate more fruits and vegetables, more whole grains, and, based on a study that came out of Harvard about the benefit of eating cooked tomatoes to reduce the risk of prostate cancer, he started eating multiple servings of cooked tomatoes per week. He also researched alternative treatments and started trying those—yoga, massage therapy, and supplements such as a vitamin B complex and saw palmetto.

But what was key was that Ben did all this in partnership with his regular doctors. His doctors understood that he wanted to wait before trying conventional therapies, but they didn't want to wait too long if it would be a risk to his health. So, they agreed on a path of watchful waiting, where Ben would be screened regularly using a prostate-specific antigen (PSA) blood test. High PSA levels would indicate the presence of prostate cancer. Whenever Ben's PSA level spiked, it was a warning sign, and he would take steps to lower his PSA level with alternative treatments.

If Ben couldn't get his PSA level down through the alternative approach, his doctors were ready to step in with more conventional treatments to prevent the cancer from growing and spreading. As Ben put it, he was keeping conventional treatments, such as radiation therapy, in his "gunny sack"—an option for when things got bad and stayed bad, despite his best efforts.

We hope Ben's story inspires you to find your own ways to incorporate complementary and alternative treatments into your treatment plan in partnership with your doctor.

Resources

The following resources may prove useful as you search for more information on complementary and alternative treatments.

National Center for Complementary and Integrative Health
Are You Considering a Complementary Health Approach?
https://nccih.nih.gov/health/decisions/consideringcam.htm

National Cancer Institute

Complementary and Alternative Medicine

https://www.cancer.gov/about-cancer/treatment/cam

National Institutes of Health

Office of Dietary Supplements

https://ods.od.nih.gov/

Mayo Clinic

Integrative Medicine: Different Techniques, One Goal

https://www.mayoclinic.org/tests-procedures/complementary
-alternative-medicine/in-depth/alternative-medicine/art
-20045267

Bandolier

Complementary and Alternative Therapies

http://www.bandolier.org.uk/booth/booths/altmed.html

NHS

Complementary and Alternative Medicine

https://www.nhs.uk/conditions/complementary-and
-alternative-medicine/

Johns Hopkins Medicine

Complementary and Alternative Medicine

https://www.hopkinsallchildrens.org/patients-families/
health-library/healthdocnew/complementary-and
-alternative-medicine-(1)

The University of Arizona

Andrew Weil Center for Integrative Medicine

https://integrativemedicine.arizona.edu/

10 | Making Tough Decisions

Dr. Abraar Karan is an internal medicine resident at Brigham and Women's Hospital and Harvard Medical School. Through his work, he's become familiar with the difficult decisions patients and their families have to make when faced with critical illness, and he often finds himself asking the question, "What am I supposed to do to be sure I'm doing the best for my patient?"

One of his many experiences battling with this question came early in his career, when he was working as an intern at a Boston-area hospital. An older man in good health had come in for a very low-risk, routine CT scan, an elective procedure done on an outpatient basis. By chance, while the man was in the CT scanner, a complication from a previous lung biopsy emerged, and his pulse unexpectedly disappeared. The hospital staff immediately jumped into action, calling out on the overhead speaker, "CODE BLUE! Ground floor imaging suite. CODE BLUE!"

Code blue is the code name hospital staff are trained to use in emergency situations when a patient is in cardiopulmonary arrest and staff need to immediately begin resuscitative efforts. While the medical team were using all of the tools at their disposal to resuscitate the patient, Dr. Karan, as the intern on duty, was tasked with making sure that the patient's code status was correct. But when he checked the patient's records, it was clear. The patient had an advance directive from six years ago that specifically stated that he did not want to be resuscitated—no exceptions.

An advance directive is a document that records a person's preferences for medical care in the event that the person is unable to communicate those decisions directly. In most cases, if there's an advance directive on file or a request to not resuscitate, it's enough to stop a medical team in their tracks. But in this case, Dr. Karan remembers the medical team struggling to agree to stop trying to save the patient's life: "Our instinct was to do everything we could to save his life. This is a man who, as of that morning, was fine. We were already midway through resuscitating him and, in that moment, we felt reasonably certain we could save him."

Dr. Karan called the patient's health proxy, the person who had been designated as the decision-maker if the patient was too incapacitated to make decisions for himself. The proxy was the patient's son, who lived in another state. "When I called to check about his father's wishes," Dr. Karan said, "the son said unequivocally, 'My father walked in there today for a CT scan, I know he would want everything done to save his life.'"

And that's exactly what the medical team did. Minutes later, the team regained the patient's pulse. He was sent to the intensive care unit and temporarily intubated on a ventilator. Within a few hours, the ventilator was removed, and the patient was on the path to recovery.

It is surprising how close Dr. Karan's patient came to a very different ending, in which the medical team would have followed what they believed were the patient's true intentions and stopped their efforts to save his life. What's even more surprising is how easily it could happen to any of us.

Thinking through Tough Decisions before Times Get Tough

We are at a remarkable time in human history where we can make important decisions about how and when we will die. But this situation brings new challenges that many of us have not thought through or prepared for.

CPR, or cardiopulmonary resuscitation, was first described in the medical literature in the 1960s.[1] It is, at its most basic, a remarkably simple series of actions that proved to be surprisingly effective. When it was introduced, many considered CPR a welcome and desired intervention with the potential to bring a person at the edge of death back to a healthy and active life. But, in reality, CPR wasn't always a welcome option. For some people, CPR didn't extend their years of healthy life, it only prolonged an uncomfortable death. As a result, the American Medical Association developed a policy outlining that people could decide if they would rather not undergo CPR. This is called a Do Not Resuscitate (DNR) order.[2]

Since then, the concept has evolved, and end-of-life planning has greatly expanded. Now, almost anytime that someone is admitted to a medical facility, even for the most mundane of reasons, they are asked about whether they would like to be resuscitated if a complication arose and they went into cardiac arrest. Doctors call this the *code status*. If you decide you want CPR in the case of a cardiac arrest, you are considered *full code*. If you only agree to certain resuscitation procedures during a medical emergency, you are *limited code*. And, if you decide you don't want to be resuscitated at all, you are *DNR*.

This is what happened with Dr. Karan's patient. Six years previously, perhaps for another intervention entirely, the patient gave an indication that he would not want to be resuscitated. That decision was critical to how he was treated all those years later.

Think Like Your Doctor: Code Status

Whether you're heading to the hospital for a relatively minor procedure or a major surgery, you need to think about your code status and how you want to be treated in the event that something goes wrong.

Thinking about our own mortality can be uncomfortable, and it can be tempting to skip past questions about how we might want to approach death, especially if we are generally healthy and there's no imminent risk. Still, we encourage you to stick with us through this chapter as it could prove useful if you are ever in that situation. It's a little bit like wearing a seatbelt—the chances of having an accident on any given car trip are low, but if it does occur, you'll be glad you wore the seatbelt.

To determine how you will choose your code status and whether you want to be resuscitated if your body fails you, first think about your own values and beliefs. Would you want death to occur naturally, whenever that happened, or would you want your life to be sustained for as long as possible? Would you be comfortable spending your final days in a hospital, or would you prefer to spend them at home? The answers may not be black and white, but knowing whether you lean more in one direction or another will help you make a more informed decision about your code status and advance directives.

The Conversation Project is a public engagement initiative that helps people think through their end-of-life wishes and talk those wishes over with their family, friends, and care team. They have created a very useful toolkit called Your Conversation Toolkit. We've included part of that toolkit at the end of this chapter, along with links to other resources, to help you think about how your values and beliefs may impact your final decision.

Another important consideration is to look at your health overall. One of the strongest predictors of the success of CPR is how healthy a person is when the cardiac arrest happens. The healthier a person is, the better their chance of survival and recovery. Another important factor is age. Young people have a better chance of survival than those who are older.

If you are like the person at the beginning of this chapter, older but in relatively good health and having a minor, elective procedure, you may want to opt for full code status, making it clear that despite any previous advance directives you may have authorized, on this day you want the medical team's full efforts to resuscitate you should anything go wrong. On the other hand, if you are being repeatedly hospitalized for an underlying progressive illness, like advanced cancer, or you are in the final stages of a degenerative disorder like amyotrophic lateral sclerosis (ALS, also known as Lou Gehrig's disease), then the chances of survival and recovery will be much lower. In addition, your underlying disease would continue to progress, and your overall health would still be in steady decline. In this case, you may feel more comfortable choosing a DNR order.

In addition to your values and overall health, you'll also want to consider the effectiveness, or lack thereof, of different forms of resuscitation, which may include CPR, medications, defibrillation, intubation, or a combination of those methods. CPR is often less effective than people think. A study of one thousand people in Michigan found that, when presented with a scenario of cardiac arrest, 72 percent of respondents expected to survive.[3] In fact, a more realistic estimate of the success rate of CPR is less than 20 percent. This misperception of the effectiveness of CPR may be due to unrealistic portrayals on television and film.[4] The reality is that less than a quarter of people who have CPR in the hospital survive to discharge. Even fewer make it to the one-year mark. And there are also side effects from the procedure. CPR can be physically traumatic, especially if you are frail, and it is not unusual to see broken ribs as a result of chest compressions.

All these factors—your values, the effectiveness and discomfort of resuscitation, and where you are on your personal health journey—should be considered when deciding on your code status. This is a choice only you can make, but it should be made thoughtfully and not on a whim as you go through the intake process on the day of your procedure at the hospital.

Though the choice is yours, there are two key points that we feel are important to mention so that you can continue to make the best decisions for your health even after you've made your choice about code status.

First, research shows that people who are DNR are less likely to receive other treatments. For example, a study of veterans with heart failure showed that those who elected DNR were less likely to receive treatments recommended by the guidelines.[5] While the DNR order very specifically refers to resuscitation, health care providers, consciously or unconsciously, seem to extend it to other treatments. From a patient's perspective, this observation is not a reason to choose either DNR or CPR. Rather, it means that extra vigilance is needed to make sure that the health care team understands the patient's preferences. Specifically, if you are DNR but still want to receive all the other appropriate treatments, it is important to mention this the first time you meet a provider so they are aware of your wishes. It may be helpful to bring this up again when treatment options are being discussed by specifically asking, "Are there other options if I was not DNR?" This type of open conversation can help reduce some of the bias that exists and ensure that each treatment decision is made on its own merit rather than being influenced by code status.

Second, many of us may feel that we would be willing to be resuscitated if we knew that we would recover and not end up on long-term life support. If this is the case for you, you may be tempted to choose a limited code, perhaps agreeing to CPR but not to being intubated. This is generally not your best option. As we've noted, even in the best of cases with a full code, CPR and other forms of resuscitation have limited effectiveness. A limited code is even less effective. There are a number of research papers on the hazards of having a limited code.[6,7] This option almost guarantees discomfort without significantly increasing your chances of survival.

A code blue works because the team is able to try a number of interrelated procedures on a patient. When the code team arrives on the scene, they have no way of knowing whether the end result will be a full recovery or complete dependence on life-support machines, like ventilators. Given this situation, if your preference is that you want to be resuscitated but not dependent on machines, then one way to achieve your goal is to be full code and appoint a health care proxy. This way, the code blue team can give you the best chance of survival using all the tools at their disposal, but should you end up completely dependent on machines, your health care proxy can make the decision to turn off life support and focus on comfort. If this approach makes sense to you, then you might consider bringing it up with your proxy and explaining that you want a time-limited trial of critical care, usually three to seven days. If things have not improved after that amount of time, then the proxy should ask the medical team to transition to comfort care. This way, you can be full code without having to commit to living on life support.

Regardless of whether or not we subscribe to this approach, all of us should consider choosing a health proxy in an effort to be prepared for the eventuality that we cannot make our own health care decisions.

Choosing a Health Proxy

Ideally, you would choose a health care proxy well before you are critically ill and with enough time to talk to them about your values, your intentions, and how you would like them to handle any decisions about your health if you're unable to do so yourself. Choose someone you trust and who is able to follow your intentions and not let their own emotions get in the way. It's okay to choose someone who is not a family member, but it may be helpful to let your family know so that when the time comes, no one is surprised.

Once you make the choice, be sure to give your proxy guidelines for decision-making, including the factors you would weigh if you could make the decision yourself. If they understand what is important to you, then they are more likely to follow through on your wishes, even if you haven't talked about specific scenarios. It also relieves them of any guilt they may feel in the process. There are a variety of tools available online that can help you with choosing a good proxy and talking about your values and desires.[8,9]

You can give your health proxy power of attorney for a specific period of time or indefinitely. You can also grant them power of attorney over certain elements of your care but not others. For example, if you live far from family and have a major surgery coming up, you may want a trusted friend who lives close by to be in the hospital acting as your proxy if things go wrong. But if your condition doesn't improve and you are incapacitated over an extended period of time, you may want to have a family member step in to make longer-term decisions about your health and your care.

The AARP, a nonprofit organization that helps people choose how they live as they age, provides state-specific advance directive forms on their website.[10] Once you've made your decision and filled out the form, it's important to make it legal and have it signed in accordance with the laws of your state or country. Sometimes this means signing the document in front of a witness, and sometimes this means having the document notarized. Even if you don't have time to have the document notarized, make sure you write down your choice of proxy and their contact information and take it with you to the hospital to share with the staff.

Even though these are difficult topics to discuss, communication is critical. As you work your way through your decision, consider bringing your primary care doctor into the discussion and let them know your reasoning. Their feedback may help you come to a final decision about what you will do. When you do come to a decision, be sure to let your primary doctor know, and let your other doctors, nurses, and care providers know your preferences.

Other End-of-Life Considerations

Whether you are contemplating CPR, DNR, or other end-of-life questions while you are young and healthy, or if you are naturally moving toward the later stages of life and these issues seem more real and relevant, there are more decisions to consider than just code status and health care proxies.

Living Wills, Advance Directives, and Physician Orders for Life-Sustaining Treatment

In the same way you might prepare a last will and testament to allocate your possessions and finances, some people decide to prepare an advance directive such as a living will to outline their preferences at the end of life. For those who have chosen a health proxy and made a decision about their code status, a living will is often unnecessary and sometimes undesirable. The story of Dr. Karan's patient at the start of this chapter is a perfect example of how advance directives can sometimes hurt more than they help. Whereas a health proxy can weigh the pros and cons of a treatment for a particular emergency against a person's wishes, an advance directive is literally black and white, with concrete, fixed orders that will apply to a broad range of situations that may not have even been a possibility when the directive was written.

That said, a living will can be useful, especially if there are certain procedures that you are sure you would not want under any circumstances. For example, some people have a religious objection to blood transfusions and would not want one even if it were lifesaving. In that case, having this clearly outlined in an advance directive can be incredibly helpful to the medical team as well as caregivers.

Physician orders for life-sustaining treatment, which are also known as medical orders for life-sustaining treatment, take the concept of advance directives to the next level. They summarize a person's wishes in the form of medical orders. This makes it quite explicit what your health care team should and should not do. On the one hand, it can provide clarity around interventions you might absolutely not want. On the other, it might be overly restrictive, and a health care proxy might be able to sort through the subtleties of care decisions more effectively.

Palliative Care and Conventional Care

As you think through end-of-life planning, it's useful to consider how and when you might consider palliative care versus conventional care. People often confuse the terms for one another, but there is a subtle yet important difference between the two. Essentially, palliative care focuses on comfort, while conventional care is focused on treating the underlying disease.

Suppose someone has end-stage heart failure and has trouble breathing because fluid is building up in their lungs. A conventional approach might involve calling 911, being admitted to a hospital, having blood tests done, receiving intravenous medications, then being admitted to an intensive care unit for around-the-clock monitoring. A palliative approach might involve a nurse coming to the house and administering oral medications to relieve discomfort from the difficulty breathing and to reduce the buildup of fluid. Notice that in the conventional approach, the intravenous medications may be administered as a stronger dose but come with the discomfort of side effects, and there may be additional follow-up needed, such as blood tests and around-the-clock monitoring. In the palliative approach, the focus is on comfort, which includes keeping the person in familiar surroundings and using oral medications, which are more comfortable and convenient than intravenous ones.

On the surface, it can seem like the palliative approach involves a lower level of care because available treatments are not being administered. This idea of somehow doing less with palliative care can be uncomfortable, but there is a landmark research study that suggests that, in some cases, less is indeed more.[11] Researchers divided patients with advanced lung cancer into two groups. One group got a consultation from the palliative care team, and the other did not. The palliative care team explained to the patients what palliative care was and provided insights to the primary care team on how to incorporate palliative options into the care of the patients. The palliative approach seemed to resonate with patients as the researchers found that they tended to forgo aggressive treatments much more so than the other group. The most impressive finding was that the palliative care group lived longer and had a better quality of life than the conventional care group.

This point is worth emphasizing—patients that chose fewer treatments lived longer. Experts believe that some of the aggressive treatments were in fact shortening life even as they attacked the underlying disease. There is increasing evidence that suggests that early involvement of the palliative care team or early referral to hospice care can improve outcomes.

Given these results, you may want to consider including some palliative care approaches alongside your conventional care if you have a disease with a poor prognosis. Thankfully, it's no longer a question of one form of care versus another. Instead, you could start with a conventional care approach with some palliative elements and, if desired, transition over time to a predominantly palliative approach. If your health care team does not offer a palliative care consultation, it might be worth asking if that option is available and how to access the service.

Hospice Care

While palliative care is a broad field in its own right, one of the most visible components of palliative care is hospice care. Hospice care is designed to support people in the very final stages of a terminal illness. This type of care may be delivered in a person's home, in a hospital, or in special inpatient hospice facilities. Inpatient facilities were created to provide people a comfortable environment at the end of life, but moving to inpatient hospice care may not be the best option for everyone. People may prefer to die in their own home, and family and friends may prefer to keep their loved ones in a familiar environment until the end.

Hospice care is sometimes less of an emotional decision for the person and their loved ones and more of a practical decision. Insurance companies usually pay for hospice care when health care providers can attest that a person's estimated survival is six months or less. Because hospice care is so expensive, whether delivered in the home or an inpatient facility, most of us are at the mercy of what our insurance companies will agree to pay for. There are numerous details regarding hospice care that are beyond the scope of this book, but if you are in this situation, we encourage you to use the wealth of information available online and some of the framing in other chapters in this book to learn as much as you can about the options that are available to you.

Caregivers

In addition to thinking about what's best for the person nearing the end of life, it's also important to think about the well-being of those caring for them. Recently, there has been increasing recognition of the burden that falls on caregivers, a burden that becomes much heavier as a person approaches the end of life. As many of us know from our own experiences, caregiving often extends well beyond physical care. Caregivers manage logistics such as schedules, appointments, housekeeping, finances, and transportation all while dealing with the emotional responsibilities of being the primary companion in many cases to the person in need.

There are many online resources that can help alleviate the burden of caregiving. A good first step is to create a care map, which is essentially a visual representation of the types of care a person may need and all the caregivers available to help provide support. Atlas of Caregiving has created a number of online tools to help you draw your map, which can be found on their website (https://atlasofcaregiving .com/). Understanding the type of care that's needed and the people available to help is the first step to expanding care for the person in need and relieving the caregiver from some of the stress, anxiety, and responsibilities of their role.

Ultimately, many of us will not get to choose the manner in which we die. However, we do have a choice in how the medical system treats us should we be unable to speak for ourselves. We are hopeful that the guidance in this chapter will help you reflect on what is important to you and give you the means to communicate your wishes to your health care team.

Tools to Help You with End-of-Life Decisions

The following text has been reproduced with permission from The Conversation Project, a public engagement initiative of the Institute for Healthcare Improvement cofounded by Pulitzer Prize winner Ellen Goodman in 2012. The goal of The Conversation Project is both simple and transformative: to have every person's wishes for end-of-life care expressed and respected.

What's most important to you as you think about how you want to live at the end of your life? What do you value most? Thinking about this will help you get ready to have the conversation.

Now finish this sentence: What matters to me at the end of life is. . .
(for example, being able to recognize my children, being in the hospital with excellent nursing care, being able to say goodbye to the ones I love)

_____

_____

_____

Sharing your "what matters to me" statement with your loved ones could be a big help down the road. It could help them communicate to your health care team what abilities are most important to you—what's worth pursuing treatment for, and what isn't.

Where I Stand Scales

Use the scales below to figure out how you want your end-of-life care to be. Select the number that best represents your feelings on the given scenario.

As a patient, I'd like to know . . .

Only the basics about my condition and my treatment				All the details about my condition and my treatment
1	**2**	**3**	**4**	**5**
O	O	O	O	O

As I receive care, I would like . . .

My health care team to do what they think is best				To have a say in every health care decision
1	**2**	**3**	**4**	**5**
O	O	O	O	O

If I had a terminal illness, I would prefer to . . .

Not know how quickly it is progressing				Know my doctor's best estimation for how long I have to live
1	**2**	**3**	**4**	**5**
O	O	O	O	O

Look at your answers. What kind of role do you want to have in the decision-making process?

_____

_____

_____

How long do you want to receive medical care?

Indefinitely, no matter how un-comfortable treatments are				Quality of life is more important to me than quantity
1	2	3	4	5
O	O	O	O	O

What are your concerns about treatment?

I'm worried that I won't get enough care				I'm worried that I'll get overly aggressive care
1	2	3	4	5
O	O	O	O	O

What are your preferences about where you want to be?

I wouldn't mind spending my last days in a health care facility				I want to spend my last days at home
1	2	3	4	5
O	O	O	O	O

Look at your answers. What do you notice about the kind of care you want to receive?

_____

_____

_____

How involved do you want your loved ones to be?

I want my loved ones to do exactly what I've said, even it makes them a little un-comfortable				I want my loved ones to do what brings them peace, even if it goes against what I've said
1	2	3	4	5
O	O	O	O	O

When it comes to your privacy . . .

When the time comes, I want to be alone				I want to be surrounded by my loved ones
1	2	3	4	5
O	O	O	O	O

When it comes to sharing information . . .

I don't want my loved ones to know everything about my health				I am comfortable with those close to me knowing everything about my health
1	2	3	4	5
O	O	O	O	O

Look at your answers. What role do you want your loved ones to play? Do you think that your loved ones know what you want, or do you think they have no idea?

_____

_____

_____

What do you feel are the three most important things that you want your friends, family, and/or health care team to understand about your wishes and preferences for end-of-life care?

1. _____

2. _____

3. _____

The full *Your Conversation Starter Kit* is available at https://thecon versationproject.org/wp-content/uploads/2017/02/Conversation Project-ConvoStarterKit-English.pdf.

Resources

Research suggests that video- and internet-based sites can facilitate a more informed decision on end-of-life directives. Here are two sites that have been studied in the literature:

> https://prepareforyourcare.org/welcome
> www.mylivingvoice.com

If you prefer a paper-based approach, you can print out some of the resources from the websites of The Conversation Project or the Coalition for Compassionate Care of California:

> https://theconversationproject.org/
> https://coalitionccc.org/tools-resources/advance-care-planning-resources/

Butler M, Ratner E, McCreedy E, Shippee N, Kane RL. Decision aids for advance care planning: an overview of the state of the science. *Annals of Internal Medicine.* 2014;161(6):408–418.

Afterword

There are many wonderful online and offline sources of health information. The downside is that they can be hard to find, and many people don't even know what to look for. Our goal with this book has been to provide guidance and context so that you can make the most of the resources available.

We wanted this book to be comprehensive and for it to include the major milestones a person encounters on their health journey. But we also didn't want it to be overwhelming. This has meant that some areas—like mental health and pregnancy—have not been discussed in depth. For those of you who are interested in digging deeper, we encourage you to delve into the references included in each chapter.

We would like to thank everyone who took the time to speak with us during the writing of the book, including those who allowed us to share their stories. We also want to acknowledge those people who have been working diligently in the field of patient empowerment, building the foundation upon which much of this work lies. The true credit belongs to them.

We are hopeful that the principles we have explored in this book and the tools we provided will help you deal more effectively with the health issues you or your loved ones are facing. We wish you the best in your search for health.

Notes

1 | The First Signs of Illness

1. To learn more about AFM, check the Centers for Disease Control and Prevention website: https://www.cdc.gov/acute-flaccid-myelitis/. You can search for scientific research on the PubMed website: https://www.ncbi.nlm.nih.gov/pubmed/.
2. The Editorial Board. An echo of polio: AFM paralyzes children and terrifies parents. *Chicago Tribune*. November 19, 2019. Available at: https://www.chicagotribune.com/opinion/editorials/ct-edit-afm-paralysis-polio-cdc-20181107-story.html. Accessed May 1, 2020.
3. Galante A, Deo P, Fox M. Polio-like Illness is on the rise with 87 possible cases. NBC News. October 12, 2018. Available at: https://www.nbcnews.com/health/health-news/cases-polio-illness-appear-be-rise-across-u-s-n919576. Accessed May 1, 2020.
4. Lannon J. How consumers find and use online health-related content in 2017. PM360. November 28, 2017. Available at: https://www.pm360online.com/how-consumers-find-and-use-online-health-related-content-in-2017/. Accessed May 1, 2020.
5. Cocco AM, Zordan R, Taylor DM, et al. Dr Google in the ED: searching for online health information by adult emergency department patients. *The Medical Journal of Australia*. 2018;209(8):342–347.
6. Fox S. The social life of health information 2011. Pew Research Center. May 12, 2011. Available at: http://www.pewinternet.org/2011/05/12/the-social-life-of-health-information-2011/. Accessed May 1, 2020.

7. Eysenbach G, Kohler Ch. What is the prevalence of health-related searches on the World Wide Web? Qualitative and quantitative analysis of search engine queries on the internet. *AMIA Annual Symposium Proceedings*. 2003:225–229.

8. Kummervold PE, Chronaki CE, Lausen B, et al. eHealth trends in Europe 2005–2007: a population-based survey. *Journal of Medical Internet Research*. 2008;10(4):e42. doi:10.2196/jmir.1023.

9. Haaland M. "Dr. Google" has wrongly convinced two in five Americans that they had a serious disease. SWNS Digital. November 8, 2019. Available at: https://www.swnsdigital.com/2019/11/dr-google-has -wrongly-convinced-two-in-five-americans-that-they-had-a-serious -disease/. Accessed May 1, 2020.

10. Zielstorff RD. Controlled vocabularies for consumer health. *Journal of Biomedical Informatics*. 2003;36(4–5):326–333.

11. White RW, Horvitz E. Cyberchondria: studies of the escalation of medical concerns in web search. *ACM Transactions on Information Systems*. 2009;27(4). doi:10.1145/1629096.1629101.

12. Lee K, Hoti K, Hughes JD, Emmerton LM. Consumer use of "Dr Google": a survey on health information-seeking behaviors and navigational needs. *Journal of Medical Internet Research*. 2015;17(12):e288. doi:10.2196/jmir.4345.

13. A review in *PLoS One* noted, "Despite the increasing pervasiveness of, and reliance on, the Internet in the area of health information, we found few reports of interventions to assist health consumers to find reliable health information online." Lee K, Hoti K, Hughes JD, Emmerton LM. Interventions to assist health consumers to find reliable online health information: a comprehensive review. *PLoS One*. 2014;9(4):e94186. doi:10.1371/journal.pone.0094186.

14. Amante DJ, Hogan TP, Pagoto SL, English TM, Lapane KL. Access to care and use of the internet to search for health information: results from the US National Health Interview Survey. *Journal of Medical Internet Research*. 2015;17(4):e106. doi:10.2196/jmir.4126.

15. Cohen G, Java R. Memory for medical history: accuracy of recall. *Applied Cognitive Psychology*. 1995;9(4):273–288. doi:10.1002 /acp.2350090402.

16. Warner MJ, Simunich TJ, Warner MK, Dado J. Use of patient-authored prehistory to improve patient experiences and accommodate federal law. *The Journal of the American Osteopathic Association*. 2017;117(2):78–84. doi:10.7556/jaoa.2017.018.

2 | Moving from Symptoms to a Diagnosis

1. We should note that Erica's story is not unusual, as many people self-diagnose gluten sensitivity. In one paper, researchers described the experiences of 147 such patients. For more details, see Biesiekierski JR, Newnham ED, Shepherd SJ, Muir JG, Gibson PR. Characterization of adults with a self-diagnosis of nonceliac gluten sensitivity. *Nutrition in Clinical Practice*. 2014:29(4):504–509.

2. To learn more about clinical reasoning, consider reading Schwartz A, Elstein AS. Clinical reasoning in medicine. In: Higgs J, Jones MA, Loftus S, Christensen N, eds. *Clinical Reasoning in the Health Professions*. 3rd ed. Boston, MA: Elsevier; 2008:223–234.

3. To learn more about differential diagnosis, you might want to read Seladi-Schulman J. What is a differential diagnosis? Healthline. Reviewed May 11, 2018. Available at: https://www.healthline.com /health/differential
-diagnosis. Accessed April 23, 2020.

4. Davis CP. Emergency department visits: we are not prepared. *The American Journal of Emergency Medicine*. 2012;30(8):1364–1370. doi:10.1016/j.ajem.2011.09.026.

5. Pincus T, Yazici Y, Swearingen CJ. Quality control of a medical history: improving accuracy with patient participation, supported by a four-page version of the multidimensional health assessment questionnaire (MDHAQ). *Rheumatics Diseases Clinics of North America*. 2009;35(4):851–860. doi:10.1016/j.rdc.2009.10.014.

6. Bell SK, Mejilla R, Anselmo M, et al. When doctors share visit notes with patients: a study of patient and doctor perceptions of documentation errors, safety opportunities and the patient-doctor relationship. *BMJ Quality & Safety*. 2017;26(4):262–270. doi:10.1136 /bmjqs-2015-004697.

7. National Academies of Sciences, Engineering, and Medicine. *Improving Diagnosis in Health Care*. Washington, DC: The National Academies Press; 2015.

8. There is a rich literature on cognitive bias in medicine. For example, see the book Groopman J. *How Doctors Think*. New York: Houghton Mifflin Harcourt; 2007.

9. Ludolph R, Schulz PJ. Debiasing health-related judgments and decision making: a systematic review. *Medical Decision Making*. 2018;38(1):3–13. doi:10.1177/0272989X17716672.

10. There are many resources that go into much more detail on how internet search engines work. For example, see the book Baeza-Yates R, Ribeiro-Neto B. *Modern Information Retrieval—the Concepts and Technology behind Search*. 2nd ed. Boston, MA: Addison Wesley; 2011.

11. Macias W, Lee M, Cunningham N. Inside the mind of the online health information searcher using think-aloud protocol. *Health Communication*. 2018;33(12):1482–1493. doi:10.1080/10410236.2017.1372040.

12. Doug Hennig has shared this story, along with many others not related to his health journey, on his personal blog: The internet (and my wife) literally saved my life. Doug Hennig. March 29, 2012. Available at: https://doughennig.blogspot.com/search?q=ankle. Accessed May 1, 2020.

Trustworthy Websites

1. A systematic review of scientific publications found that the most commonly used criteria to determine the reliability of a website were the identity of site owners, consensus among multiple sources, the use of professional medical terms and technical vocabularies, and limited advertisements: Yalin S, Zhang Y, Gwizdka J, Trace CB. Consumer evaluation of the quality of online health information: systematic literature review of relevant criteria and indicators. *Journal of Medical Internet Research*. 2019;21(5):e12522. A study from Florida summarized a similar set of criteria into the acronym GATOR (Genuine, Accurate, Trustworthy, Originates from a reliable source, and is Readable): Weber BA, Derrico DJ, Yoon SL, Sherwill-Navarro P. Educating patients to evaluate web-based health care information: the GATOR approach to healthy surfing. *Journal of Clinical Nursing*. 2010;19(9-10):1371–1377.

2. Semigran HL, Linder JA, Gidengil C, Mehrotra A. Evaluation of symptom checkers for self diagnosis and triage: audit study. *BMJ*. 2015;351:h3480.

3. Chambers D, Cantrell AJ, Johnson M, et al. Digital and online symptom checkers and health assessment/triage services for urgent health problems: systematic review. *BMJ Open*. 2019;9(8):e027743.

Other Places to Turn beyond the Internet

1. Coombs B. Health-care insurers are beefing up their apps to make you like them more. CNBC. Published January 27, 2018. Updated January 29, 2018. Available at: https://www.cnbc.com/2018/01/26/health-care -insurers-are-beefing-up-their-apps-to-make-you-like-them-more.html. Accessed May 1, 2020.

3 | Meeting with Your Doctor about Your Diagnosis

1. Shapiro J, Yu R, White MK. Conflicting doctor and patient agendas: a case illustration. *Journal of Clinical Outcomes Management.* 2000;7(10):41–46.
2. National Academies of Sciences, Engineering, and Medicine. *Improving Diagnosis in Health Care.* Washington, DC: National Academies Press; 2015.
3. Glaser E. Changing chronic disease primary care patients' participation through web training: does it make a difference? Published 2018. Available at: https://www.semanticscholar.org/paper/Changing-chronic -disease-primary-care-patients'-web-Glaser/98880eff61762dd207f c3e221dc3863f73ef9409#paper-header. Accessed April 26, 2020.
4. D'Agostino TA, Atkinson TM, Latella LE, et al. Promoting patient participation in healthcare interactions through communication skills training: a systematic review. *Patient Education and Counseling.* 2017;100(7):1247–1257. doi:10.1016/j.pec.2017.02.016.
5. Bussey L. *The Use and Integration of Online Information in Health Decision Making.* [dissertation]. Newcastle upon Tyne, UK: Northumbria University; 2018.
6. Several studies have shown the benefit of a patient agenda: Anderson MO, Jackson SL, Oster NV, et al. Patients typing their own visit agendas into an electronic medical record: pilot in a safety-net clinic. *Annals of Family Medicine.* 2017;15(2):158–161. doi:10.1370 /afm.2036. Middleton JF, McKinley RK, Gillies CL. Effect of patient completed agenda forms and doctors' education about the agenda on the outcome of consultations: randomised controlled trial. *BMJ.* 2006;332(7552):1238–1242. However, there is some variation within the literature, and some studies, like this one, did not show a benefit: Early F, Everden AJ, O'Brien CM, Fagan PL, Fuld JP. Patient agenda setting in respiratory outpatients: a randomized

controlled trial. *Chronic Respiratory Disease*. 2015;12(4):347–356. doi:10.1177/1479972315598696. Overall, though, we believe that having a patient agenda can be beneficial to patients, and it certainly can't hurt.

7. During your appointment. Agency for Healthcare Research and Quality. Content last reviewed September 2012. Available at: https://www.ahrq.gov/patients-consumers/patient-involvement/ask-your-doctor/questions-during-appointment.html. Accessed April 26, 2020.

8. Kessels RP. Patients' memory for medical information. *Journal of the Royal Society of Medicine*. 2003;96(5):219–222.

9. Laws MB, Lee Y, Taubin T, Rogers WH, Wilson IB. Factors associated with patient recall of key information in ambulatory specialty care visits: results of an innovative methodology. *PLoS One*. 2018;13(2):e0191940. doi:10.1371/journal.pone.0191940.

10. Tsulukidze M, Durand MA, Barr PJ, Mead T, Elwyn G. Providing recording of clinical consultation to patients—a highly valued but underutilized intervention: a scoping review. *Patient Education and Counseling*. 2014;95(3):297–304. doi:10.1016/j.pec.2014.02.007.

11. Some states have laws that require both parties' consent to recording a conversation, which means that secretly recording a visit without the doctor's consent could be illegal.

12. Davis C. What is teach-back? Institute for Healthcare Improvement. Available at: http://www.ihi.org/education/IHIOpenSchool/resources/Pages/AudioandVideo/ConnieDavis-WhatIsTeachBack.aspx. Accessed January 2, 2020.

13. Judson TJ, Detsky AS, Press MJ. Encouraging patients to ask questions: how to overcome "white-coat silence." *JAMA*. 2013;309(22):2325–2326. doi:10.1001/jama.2013.5797.

14. Salisbury H. Helen Salisbury: the informed patient. *BMJ*. 2019;364:l638. doi:10.1136/bmj.l638.

15. Green-Hopkins I. Search at your own risk: online health queries and your patient. *The Journal of Emergency Medicine*. 2019;57(4):571–572. doi:10.1016/j.jemermed.2019.06.044.

16. Bussey L, Sillence E. (How) do people negotiate online information into their decision making with healthcare professionals? Proceedings of the 2017 International Conference on Digital Health; July 2–5, 2017; London, UK.

17. O'Sullivan JW, Albasri A, Nicholson BD, et al. Overtesting and undertesting in primary care: a systematic review and meta-analysis. *BMJ Open*. 2018;8(2):e018557. doi:10.1136/bmjopen-2017-018557.

18. Schulte F. How a urine test after back surgery triggered a $17,850 bill. NPR. February 16, 2018. Available at: https://www.npr.org/sections/health-shots/2018/02/16/584296663/how-a-urine-test-after-back-surgery-triggered-a-17-800-bill. Accessed April 26, 2020.

19. CPT code stands for Current Procedural Terminology code. It is a medical code set maintained by the American Medical Association. It helps keep everyone on the same page about the exact test that is ordered so that the lab or imaging facility does the correct test and the insurance company pays the appropriate amount.

4 | Receiving a Diagnosis

1. Halsey's tearful acceptance speech from the 2018 Blossom Ball. Endometriosis Foundation of America. Posted March 20, 2018. Available at: https://www.endofound.org/watch-and-read-halseys-tearful-acceptance-speech-from-the-2018-blossom-ball. Accessed April 26, 2020.

2. How to prepare for a doctor's appointment. National Institute on Aging. Content reviewed February 3, 2020. Available at: https://www.nia.nih.gov/health/how-prepare-doctors-appointment. Accessed April 26, 2020.

3. de Luca R, Patrizia D, Cinzia G, Gianluca LC, Giuseppe C. The patient-physician relationship in the face of oncological disease: a review of literature on the emotional and psychological reactions of patients and physician. *Acta Medica Mediterranea*. 2016;32(6):1827–1833. doi:10.19193/0393-6384_2016_6_170.

4. National Academies of Sciences, Engineering, and Medicine. *Improving Diagnosis in Health Care*. Washington, DC: National Academies Press; 2015.

5. Jerrard J. "A hospitalist saved my life." *The Hospitalist*. 2005 June;2005(6). Available at: https://www.the-hospitalist.org/hospitalist/article/123026/hospitalist-saved-my-life. Accessed May 1, 2020.

6. The literature is summarized in this article: Carroll AE. To be sued less, doctors should consider talking to patients more. *The New York Times*. June 1, 2015. Available at: https://www.nytimes.com/2015/06/02/upshot/to-be-sued-less-doctors-should-talk-to-patients-more.html. Accessed May 1, 2020.

7. van Dalen I, Groothoff J, Stewart R, Spreeuwenberg P, Groenewegen P, van Horn J. Motives for seeking a second opinion in orthopaedic surgery. *Journal of Health Services Research & Policy*. 2001;6(4):195–201.

8. Sikora K. Second opinions for patients with cancer. *BMJ*. 1995;311(7014):1179–1180. doi:https://doi.org/10.1136/bmj.311.7014.1179.

9. Office for Civil Rights. *Your Health Information Privacy Rights*. Available at: https://www.hhs.gov/sites/default/files/ocr/privacy/hipaa/understanding/consumers/consumer_rights.pdf. Accessed April 26, 2020.

10. How to understand your lab results. MedlinePlus. Page last updated February 25, 2020. Page last reviewed August 16, 2018. Available at: https://medlineplus.gov/lab-tests/how-to-understand-your-lab-results/. Accessed April 26, 2020.

11. McCarthy M. US doctors are judged more on bedside manner than effectiveness of care, survey finds. *BMJ*. 2014;349:g4864. doi:10.1136/bmj.g4864.

12. Morche J, Mathes T, Pieper D. Relationship between surgeon volume and outcomes: a systematic review of systematic reviews. *Systematic Reviews*. 2016;5(1):204.

13. Greenfield G, Pliskin JS, Feder-Bubis P, Wientroub S, Davidovitch N. Patient-physician relationships in second opinion encounters–the physicians' perspective. *Social Science & Medicine*. 2012;75(7):1202–1212. doi:10.1016/j.socscimed.2012.05.026.

14. Meyer AN, Longhurst CA, Singh H. Crowdsourcing diagnosis for patients with undiagnosed illnesses: an evaluation of CrowdMed. *Journal of Medical Internet Research*. 2016;18(1):e12. doi:10.2196/jmir.4887.

15. Juusola JL, Quisel TR, Foschini L, Ladapo JA. The impact of an online crowdsourcing diagnostic tool on health care utilization: a case study using a novel approach to retrospective claims analysis. *Journal of Medical Internet Research*. 2016;18(6):e127. doi:10.2196/jmir.5644.

16. Nobles AL, Leas EC, Althouse BM, et al. Requests for diagnoses of sexually transmitted diseases on a social media platform. *JAMA*. 2019;322(17):1712–1713. doi:10.1001/jama.2019.14390.

Professional Health Advocates

1. Interview and hire a patient advocate in 4 easy steps. The AdvoConnection Directory. Available at: https://advoconnection.com/hire-a-patient-advocate/. Accessed May 1, 2020.

5 | Deciding on Treatment

1. For more background on goal-directed care, see this paper: Reuben DB, Tinetti ME. Goal-oriented patient care—an alternative health outcomes paradigm. *The New England Journal of Medicine*. 2012;366 (9):777–779. doi:10.1056/NEJMp1113631. You can also find more information in this book: Mold JW. *Achieving Your Personal Health Goals: A Patient's Guide*. Chapel Hill, NC: Full Court Press; 2017.

2. Tinetti ME, Naik AD, Dodson JA. Moving from disease-centered to patient goals–directed care for patients with multiple chronic conditions: patient value-based care. *JAMA Cardiology*. 2016;1(1):9–10. doi:10.1001/jamacardio.2015.0248.

3. Rosenhek R, Rader F, Klaar U, et al. Outcome of watchful waiting in asymptomatic severe mitral regurgitation. *Circulation*. 2006;113(18): 2238–2244.

4. Llor C, Bjerrum L. Antimicrobial resistance: risk associated with antibiotic overuse and initiatives to reduce the problem. *Therapeutic Advances in Drug Safety*. 2014;5(6):229–241. doi:10.1177/2042098614 554919.

5. Rosenberg W, Donald A. Evidence based medicine: an approach to clinical problem-solving. *BMJ*. 1995;310(6987):1122–1126.

6. Lenzer J. Why we can't trust clinical guidelines. *BMJ*. 2013;346:f3830. doi:10.1136/bmj.f3830.

7. Siemieniuk R, Guyatt G. What is GRADE? BMJ Best Practice. Available at: https://bestpractice.bmj.com/info/toolkit/learn-ebm/what-is -grade/. Accessed April 26, 2020.

8. Kenefick H, Lee J, Fleishman V. *Improving Physician Adherence to Clinical Practice Guidelines: Barriers and Strategies for Change*. Cambridge, MA: New England Healthcare Institute; February 2008.

9. Barth JH, Misra S, Aakre KM, et al. Why are clinical practice guidelines not followed? *Clinical Chemistry and Laboratory Medicine*. 2016;54(7):1133–1139. doi:10.1515/cclm-2015-0871.

6 | Medications

1. Whit. My journey to seizure control. Changing Focus: Epilepsy. Available at: http://www.cf-epilepsy.com/my-journey-to-seizure-control/. Accessed April 26, 2020.

2. Martin K, Jackson CF, Levy RG, Cooper PN. Ketogenic diet and other dietary treatments for epilepsy. *The Cochrane Database of Systematic Reviews*. 2016;2:CD001903. doi:10.1002/14651858.CD001903.pub3.

3. Hamd RS, Hasbini DA. Adolescent's hair loss due to levetiracetam. *Journal of Pediatric Epilepsy*. 2018;07(04):152–153. doi:10.1055/s-0038-1666814.

4. Barry MJ, Edgman-Levitan S. Shared decision making—pinnacle of patient-centered care. *The New England Journal of Medicine*. 2012;366(9):780–781. doi:10.1056/NEJMp1109283.

5. Drug and Therapeutics Bulletin. An introduction to patient decision aids. *BMJ*. 2013;347:f4147. doi:10.1136/bmj.f4147.

6. Kardas P, Lewek P, Matyjaszczyk M. Determinants of patient adherence: a review of systematic reviews. *Frontiers in Pharmacology*. 2013;4:91. doi:10.3389/fphar.2013.00091.

7. Kripalani S, Yao X, Haynes RB. Interventions to enhance medication adherence in chronic medical conditions: a systematic review. *Archives of Internal Medicine*. 2007;167(6):540–550.

8. Britten N. Medication errors: the role of the patient. *British Journal of Clinical Pharmacology*. 2009;67(6):646–650. doi:10.1111/j.1365-2125.2009.03421.x.

9. Van Nuys K, Joyce G, Ribero R, Goldman DP. *Overpaying for Prescription Drugs: The Copay Clawback Phenomenon*. Los Angeles, CA: USC Leonard D. Schaeffer Center for Health Policy & Economics; March 2018.

10. How to buy medicines safely from an online pharmacy. US Food & Drug Administration. Content current as of January 25, 2018. Available at: https://www.fda.gov/consumers/consumer-updates/how-buy-medicines-safely-online-pharmacy. Accessed April 26, 2020.

7 | Surgery

1. Leilani L. I'm not letting my fear of surgery control my life. Muscular Dystrophy News Today. Published August 6, 2019. Available at: https://musculardystrophynews.com/2019/08/06/surgery-gallbladder-gallstones-malignant-hyperthermia/. Accessed April 27, 2020.

2. For more information, visit http://decisionaid.ohri.ca/AZlist.html.

3. Sacks GD, Dawes AJ, Ettner SL, et al. Surgeon perception of risk and

benefit in the decision to operate. *Annals of Surgery*. 2016;264(6):896–903.

4. Bozic KJ, Belkora J, Chan V, et al. Shared decision making in patients with osteoarthritis of the hip and knee: results of a randomized controlled trial. *The Journal of Bone and Joint Surgery. American Volume*. 2013;95(18):1633–1639. doi:10.2106/JBJS.M.00004.

5. Morche J, Mathes T, Pieper D. Relationship between surgeon volume and outcomes: a systematic review of systematic reviews. *Systematic Reviews*. 2016;5(1):204.

6. For more information, see https://projects.propublica.org/surgeons.

7. For more information, see https://www.checkbook.org/surgeon ratings/.

8. For more information, see https://www.medicare.gov/hospital compare.

9. For more information, see https://www.leapfroggroup.org/ compare-hospitals.

10. The available research suggests that facilities that do more procedures have better outcomes, but this is not so ironclad that you have to find a center with a minimum volume. See Lillemoe KD. Surgical volume/ outcome debate. *Annals of Surgery*. 2017;265(2):270. doi:10.1097/ SLA.0000000000002110.

11. Sindhupakorn B, Numpaisal PO, Thienpratharn S, Jomkoh D. A home visit program versus a non-home visit program in total knee replacement patients: a randomized controlled trial. *Journal of Orthopaedic Surgery and Research*. 2019;14(1):405. doi:10.1186/s13018-019-1412-6.

12. Saint S. Hand washing stops infections, so why do health care workers skip it? Institute for Healthcare Policy & Innovation. Published May 18, 2016. Available at: https://ihpi.umich.edu/news/hand -washing-stops-infections-so-why-do-health-care-workers-skip-it. Accessed April 27, 2020.

13. Fernandes Agreli H, Murphy M, Creedon S, et al. Patient involvement in the implementation of infection prevention and control guidelines and associated interventions: a scoping review. *BMJ Open*. 2019;9(3): e025824. doi:10.1136/bmjopen-2018-025824.

8 | Lifestyle Treatment Options

1. Arena R, McNeil A, Sagner M, Hills AP. The current global state of key lifestyle characteristics: health and economic implications. *Progress in Cardiovascular Diseases*. 2017;59(5):422–429. doi:10.1016/j.pcad.2017.02.002.

2. Benziger CP, Roth GA, Moran AE. The Global Burden of Disease study and the preventable burden of NCD. *Global Heart*. 2016;11(4):393–397. doi:10.1016/j.gheart.2016.10.024.

3. Anderson L, Oldridge N, Thompson DR, et al. Exercise-based cardiac rehabilitation for coronary heart disease: Cochrane systematic review and meta-analysis. *Journal of the American College of Cardiology*. 2016;67(1):1–12. doi:10.1016/j.jacc.2015.10.044.

4. Kullo IJ, Rooke TW. Clinical practice. Peripheral artery disease. *The New England Journal of Medicine*. 2016;374(9):861–871. doi:10.1056/NEJMcp1507631.

5. Bartsch AL, Härter M, Niedrich J, Brütt AL, Buchholz A. A systematic literature review of self-reported smoking cessation counseling by primary care physicians. *PLoS One*. 2016;11(12):e0168482. doi:10.1371/journal.pone.0168482.

6. Graham AL, Amato MS. Twelve million smokers look online for smoking cessation help annually: Health Information National Trends Survey data, 2005–2017. *Nicotine & Tobacco Research*. 2019;21(2):249–252. doi:10.1093/ntr/nty043.

7. Saneei P, Salehi-Abargouei A, Esmaillzadeh A, Azadbakht L. Influence of Dietary Approaches to Stop Hypertension (DASH) diet on blood pressure: a systematic review and meta-analysis on randomized controlled trials. *Nutrition, Metabolism, and Cardiovascular Diseases*. 2014;24(12):1253–1261. doi:10.1016/j.numecd.2014.06.008.

8. Salehi-Abargouei A, Maghsoudi Z, Shirani F, Azadbakht L. Effects of Dietary Approaches to Stop Hypertension (DASH)-style diet on fatal or nonfatal cardiovascular diseases—incidence: a systematic review and meta-analysis on observational prospective studies. *Nutrition*. 2013;29(4):611–618. doi:10.1016/j.nut.2012.12.018.

9. McAfee T, Babb S, McNabb S, Fiore MC. Helping smokers quit—opportunities created by the Affordable Care Act. *The New England Journal of Medicine*. 2015;372(1):5–7. doi:10.1056/NEJMp1411437.

10. Lindström D, Sadr Azodi O, Wladis A, et al. Effects of a perioperative

smoking cessation intervention on postoperative complications: a randomized trial. *Annals of Surgery.* 2008;248(5):739–745. doi:10.1097 /SLA.0b013e3181889d0d.

11. Hughes MJ, Hackney RJ, Lamb PJ, Wigmore SJ, Christopher Deans DA, Skipworth RJE. Prehabilitation before major abdominal surgery: a systematic review and meta-analysis. *World Journal of Surgery.* 2019;43(7):1661–1668. doi:10.1007/s00268-019-04950-y.

12. Zadrozny B. Parents are poisoning their children with bleach to "cure" autism. These moms are trying to stop it. NBCNews. May 21, 2019. Available at: https://www.nbcnews.com/tech/internet/moms-go -undercover-fight-fake-autism-cures-private-facebook-groups -n1007871. Accessed April 30, 2020.

13. For more information, see https://www.cdc.gov/diabetes/prevention /program-providers.htm.

14. Williams RB. Cardiology patient page. Depression after heart attack: why should I be concerned about depression after a heart attack? *Circulation.* 2011;123(25):e639–e640. doi:10.1161/CIRCULATION AHA.110.017285.

15. Erogul M. The perils of being your own doctor. *The Guardian.* August 4, 2016. Available at: https://www.theguardian.com/news/2016 /aug/04/perils-being-your-own-doctor-als. Accessed April 30, 2020.

16. Wang PS, Angermeyer M, Borges G, et al. Delay and failure in treatment seeking after first onset of mental disorders in the World Health Organization's World Mental Health Survey Initiative. *World Psychiatry.* 2007;6(3):177–185.

17. Reblin M, Uchino BN. Social and emotional support and its implication for health. *Current Opinion in Psychiatry.* 2008;21(2):201–205. doi:10.1097/YCO.0b013e3282f3ad89.

18. Bove R. Social media in the age of the "new polio". *The New England Journal of Medicine.* 2019;380(13):1195–1197. doi:10.1056/NEJM p1813390.

19. Smailhodzic E, Hooijsma W, Boonstra A, Langley DJ. Social media use in healthcare: a systematic review of effects on patients and on their relationship with healthcare professionals. *BMC Health Services Research.* 2016;16:442. doi:10.1186/s12913-016-1691-0.

9 | Complementary and Alternative Treatments

1. Ng JY, Boon HS, Thompson AK, Whitehead CR. Making sense of "alternative," "complementary," "unconventional" and "integrative" medicine: exploring the terms and meanings through a textual analysis. *BMC Complementary and Alternative Medicine*. 2016;16:134. doi:10.1186/s12906-016-1111-3.

2. Harris P, Rees R. The prevalence of complementary and alternative medicine use among the general population: a systematic review of the literature. *Complementary Therapies in Medicine*. 2000;8(2):88–96.

3. Nguyen T, Karl M, Santini A. Red yeast rice. *Foods*. 2017;6(3):E19. doi:10.3390/foods6030019.

4. How red yeast rice lowers your cholesterol. Dr. Sam Robbins. Available at: https://www.drsamrobbins.com/cholesterol/how-red-yeast-rice -lowers-your-cholesterol/. Accessed April 30, 2020.

5. Loubser L, Weider KI, Drake SM. Acute liver injury induced by red yeast rice supplement. *BMJ Case Reports*. 2019;12(3):e227961. doi:10.1136/bcr-2018-227961.

6. Farkouh A, Baumgärtel C. Mini-review: medication safety of red yeast rice products. *International Journal of General Medicine*. 2019;12:167–171. doi:10.2147/IJGM.S202446.

7. White NJ, Hien TT, Nosten FH. A brief history of qinghaosu. *Trends in Parasitology*. 2015;31(12):607–610. doi:10.1016/j.pt.2015.10.010.

8. To learn more about how to read a scientific paper, visit https://www .understandinghealthresearch.org/useful-information/how-to-read-a -scientific-paper-4 or read Harris M, Taylor J, Jackson D. *Clinical Evidence Made Easy: The Basics of Evidence-Based Medicine*. Surrey, UK: Scion Publishing Limited; 2014.

9. Foley H, Steel A. Patient perceptions of clinical care in complementary medicine: a systematic review of the consultation experience. *Patient Education and Counseling*. 2017;100(2):212–223. doi:10.1016 /j.pec.2016.09.015.

10. Jou J, Johnson PJ. Nondisclosure of complementary and alternative medicine use to primary care physicians: findings from the 2012 National Health Interview Survey. *JAMA Internal Medicine*. 2016;176(4):545–546. doi:10.1001/jamainternmed.2015.8593.

11. Nahin RL, Barnes PM, Stussman BJ. Expenditures on complementary health approaches: United States, 2012. *National Health Statistics Reports*. 2016;(95):1–11.

12. Harvard Prostate Knowledge. A patient's story: why one man opted for lifestyle changes instead of treatment. Harvard Health Publishing. Posted November 10, 2009. Available at: https://www.health.harvard.edu/blog/a-patients-story-why-one-man-opted-for-lifestyle-changes-instead-of-treatment-2009111012. Accessed April 30, 2020.

10 | Making Tough Decisions

1. Kouwenhoven WB, Jude JR, Knickerbocker GG. Closed-chest cardiac massage. *JAMA*. 1960;173:1064–1067.
2. Rabkin MT, Gillerman G, Rice NR. Orders not to resuscitate. *The New England Journal of Medicine*. 1976;295(7):364–366.
3. Ouellette L, Puro A, Weatherhead J, et al. Public knowledge and perceptions about cardiopulmonary resuscitation (CPR): results of a multicenter survey. *The American Journal of Emergency Medicine*. 2018;36(10):1900–1901. doi:10.1016/j.ajem.2018.01.103.
4. Portanova J, Irvine K, Yi JY, Enguidanos S. It isn't like this on TV: revisiting CPR survival rates depicted on popular TV shows. *Resuscitation*. 2015;96:148–150. doi:10.1016/j.resuscitation.2015.08.002.
5. Chen JL, Sosnov J, Lessard D, Goldberg RJ. Impact of do-not-resuscitation orders on quality of care performance measures in patients hospitalized with acute heart failure. *American Heart Journal*. 2008;156(1):78–84. doi:10.1016/j.ahj.2008.01.030.
6. Sanders A, Schepp M, Baird M. Partial do-not-resuscitate orders: a hazard to patient safety and clinical outcomes? *Critical Care Medicine*. 2011;39(1):14–18. doi:10.1097/CCM.0b013e3181feb8f6.
7. Zapata JA, Widera E. Partial codes-a symptom of a larger problem. *JAMA Internal Medicine*. 2016;176(8):1058–1059. doi:10.1001/jamainternmed.2016.2540.
8. Institute for Healthcare Improvement, The Conversation Project. *Who Will Speak for You? How to Choose and Be a Health Care Proxy*. The Conversation Project; 2019. Available at: https://theconversationproject.org/wp-content/uploads/2017/03/ConversationProject-Proxy-Kit-English.pdf. Accessed April 30, 2020.
9. Institute for Healthcare Improvement, The Conversation Project. *Your Conversation Starter Kit: When it Comes to End-of-Life Care, Talking Matters*. The Conversation Project; 2019. Available at: https://thecon

169

versationproject.org/wp-content/uploads/2017/02/Conversation
Project-ConvoStarterKit-English.pdf. Accessed April 30, 2020.

10. Advance directive forms. AARP. Updated February 25, 2020. Available
at: https://www.aarp.org/caregiving/financial-legal/free-printable
-advance-directives/. Accessed April 30, 2020.

11. Temel JS, Greer JA, Muzikansky A, et al. Early palliative care for
patients with metastatic non-small-cell lung cancer. *The New England
Journal of Medicine*. 2010;363(8):733–742. doi:10.1056/NEJMoa
1000678.

Index

Index

Index